Kissing Frogs

Practical Uses of Hypnotherapy

Chaplain Paul G. Durbin, Ph.D.

KENDALL/HUNT PUBLISHING COMPANY
4050 Westmark Drive Dubuque, Iowa 52002

ISBN 0-7872-1934-7

Library of Congress Catalog Card Number: 95-82137

Printed in the United States of America
10 9 8 7 6 5 4 3 2 1

Dedication

Over the years many people have touched my life and each has contributed to who I am today. I dedicate this book to all of them but a few I wish to acknowledge by name. My Dad, Reverend B. Paul Durbin (1903-1983) taught me to never stop learning and to acquire my own faith expression. My mom, Annie B. Durbin-Pullig taught me to be honest and to respect others. My wife, Bobbie has supported me with her friendship and love since 1958.

Others I would like to recognize are my sons, Timothy Paul and his wife Shannon, and Scott Kimball and his wife Gretchen; my stepfather, Mr. Gordon Pullig; my Associate Chaplain Judy Nelson; my secretaries, Kim Purdum and Terri Kirn; the administrative, medical staff, employees, and patients of Pendleton Memorial Methodist Hospital, Leslie Longaçre, R.D. Longacre, Chaplain Ray Stephens and you who read this book.

December 5, 1995

Dear Chaplain Durbin:

I just wanted to thank you for the hypnosis sessions you conducted during my pregnancy to help allay my anxiety regarding claustrophobic feelings. On October 16 I delivered a healthy 7 lb. 11 oz. baby boy—Cooper Matthew. The relaxation techniques you taught me were very helpful and the duration of my pregnancy after our sessions was free of anxiety as was my labor and delivery. Thank you again for all your help.

Fondly,

Colleen Brahney Lemsine

Contents

Foreword by R.D. Longacre, Ph.D., F.B.H.A.

In my thirty years of professional practice as an allied health care educator and complementary medicine provider I have emphasized the need to understand concepts rather than simply memorizing formulas, facts, published data and self-help therapy techniques. Chaplain Durbin attended a class I presented several years ago and immediately distinguished himself as a conceptual scholar as well as a seasoned counselor who helped his clients by asking the question, "Why not?"—rather than questioning them about why they could or why they could not.

As the Administrator for the National Board of Hypnotherapy and Hypnotic Anesthesiology, I have had the privilege of working with Dr. Durbin at Board Meetings and Educational Planning Sessions. I continue to be amazed at his ability to look at a problem and find a solution by first asking, "Why not?" This practical approach to problem solving and Pastoral counseling is the subliminal message between every line of this book.

While I was reviewing the manuscript for this book in preparation for writing the foreword, my ten-year-old daughter walked into my office and looked at the title page. "Is this a book about how to kiss frogs?" she said. "No, it is a book about learning to understand and love yourself and make good things happen in your life," I replied. She stood silently for a moment and then informed me, "Kids say that holding a frog will give you warts. But I think that if you kiss a frog it will love you and become a friend." After her pronouncement of wisdom that only a ten-year-old little girl can understand, she left the room saying, "Friends can't give you warts Dad and frogs won't give you warts if you make friends with them first."

Kissing Frogs is a book about making friends. Making friends with the mental, spiritual and physical components inside of you that create what Dr. Durbin refers to as the Human Trinity. *Kissing Frogs* is a book about healing the tranquility that is normal and naturally created within everyone when they ask the question, "Why not?"

Through the use of case studies, healing stories and easy to understand self-help techniques, Dr. Durbin takes the mystery and superstition out of the clinical application of visualization and guided imagery as a tool for pastoral or personal counseling. He outlines clinical and educational experiences that are benchmarks of learning for all licensed health care professionals.

This book has a pattern of words that read more like music than printed thoughts on a page. As I read page after page, I am reminded of the lyrics of a song by a popular recording artist. In a portion of her song, "Seeds," Kathy Mattea says, "In God's hands we start the same, but where we land is sometimes fertile soil sometimes sand. We are all just seeds in God's hands. As I'm standing at a crossroads once again, I'm reminded we're all the same when we begin and in the end, we're all just seeds in God's hands."

You do not have to be a Christian or a believer in God to benefit from the teaching stories and self-help techniques presented in this book in an easy to understand and enjoyable reading style.

I was flattered when Dr. Durbin asked me to write the forward to his first book, *Human Trinity Hypnotherapy.* At that time I accurately predicted that his first contribution to the library of published works in the area of the art and science of hypnotherapy would become a best seller among his peers and serious professionals of holistic health and complementary medicine. Kissing Frogs is a natural evolution of his first work that will be much sought after by serious scholars, graduate students and all of those who wish to utilize the abilities of their mind to achieve a more abundant life.

I urge you to set aside a special time in your life and enjoy this magical work of love, hope and miracles to its fullest.

DR. R.D. LONGACRE

Dr. Longacre is a Diplomat of the American Institute of Hypnotherapy and a Fellow of the National Board of Hypnotherapy and Hypnotic Anesthesiology. He is the author of *Client-Centered Hypnotherapy* and *Visualization and Guided Imagery for Pain Management* (both published by Kendall/Hunt in 1995), six other textbooks and numerous articles about hypnotherapy and hypnotic anesthesiology for pain management. Dr. Longacre is a past president and member of the board of directors of the California Council of Hypnotherapy, American Board of Hypnotherapy, National Society of Hypnotherapists and the American Association of Catastrophic Illness Counselors. He currently serves as the Administrator for the National Board of Hypnotherapy and Hypnotic Anesthesiology.

About the Author

Chaplain Paul G. Durbin is a United Methodist Minister serving as Director of Pastoral Care at Pendleton Memorial Methodist Hospital in New Orleans, Louisiana. He has been on Pendleton Memorial Methodist Hospital staff since 1975 and has been Director since 1982. He is a retired Military Chaplain who last served as Army National Guard Special Assistant to the Chief of Chaplain, Army with rank of Brigadier General.

Chaplain Durbin has a Bachelor of Arts Degree from Centenary College of Louisiana; a Master of Divinity from Emory University, Atlanta, Georgia; Ph.D. from the American Institute of Hypnotherapy, Irvine, California; and has completed four quarters of Clinical Pastoral Education at Walter Reed A.M.C., Washington, D.C.

He is a member of the College of Chaplains, the Louisiana Chaplain Association, and the International Association of Counselors and Therapists. He is a certified Clinical Hypnotherapist with the American Association of Professional Hypnotherapists, National Association of Clergy Hypnotherapists, American Council of Hypnotist Examiners, National Board of Hypnotherapy and Hypnotic Anesthesiology, the National Society of Clinical Hypnotherapists, National Guild of Hypnotists and International Medical and Dental Hypnotherapy Association. He is President and Diplomat with NACH. He is a Fellow with AAPH and NBHA. He is on the Board of NACH, NBHA, and the IMDHA. In 1986-87, he was "Member of the Year" with NACH. He received the NBHA "Professional Excellency" Award for 1991 and the "Pen and Quill" Award in 1992 and Honorary Service Award from IMDHA in 1992. Upon receipt of the IHHF Sealah Award for Hypnotherapy, Chaplain Durbin was inducted into the International Hypnosis Hall of Fame in March 1992.

Chaplain Durbin has written a number of articles and conducted numerous seminars throughout the nation on Pastoral Care, Stress Management, Ethical Consideration of Life Support Systems, Dying and Grief and Hypnotherapy. Chaplain Durbin teaches courses on "Hypnosis" at Nunez Community College in Chalmette, Louisiana. He has authored a booklet, "Introduction to the Value of Hypnosis," published by Pendleton Memorial Methodist Hospital Print Shop and a book, *Human Trinity Hypnotherapy,* published by Access Publishing, Ann Arbor, Michigan, for which he received the 1994 Pen and Quill award from NBHA.

PREFACE

Kissing Frogs: The Practical Use of Hypnotherapy puts into practice the theories of my first book, *Human Trinity Hypnotherapy.* I have not used footnotes in this book because most of the chapters were taken from seminars or lectures. I do give credit to those who have influenced me in the bibliographies. A bibliography follows some chapters and the book concludes with an extensive bibliography which includes books, video and audio tapes.

I would like to recognize some individuals who have influenced me either by their writings, seminars, tapes, or personal conversations: A.M. Krasner, A.M. Wolff, R.D. "Sean" Longacre, Bill Curtis, Art Winkler, J.A. "Mach" McMurtrey, Albert Bottari, Gordon Boyd, Sol Lewis, Louis Bauer, Anthony Caito, Ormand McGill, Cherylanne Atwood, Ann Spencer, Daniel Zalling, John Kappas, Patty McCormick, and hundreds of others.

Section One, "Contributions to Human Trinity Hypnotherapy," recognizes individuals outside the field of hypnotherapy whose works have contributed to my understanding of human nature. A case history follows each chapter to demonstrate the use of hypnotherapy using techniques developed from my understanding of the contributor. Section Two, "Review and Update of Human Trinity Hypnotherapy," contains case histories, manuscripts of seminars, lectures, articles, and writings. Section Three, "Case Histories" demonstrates my therapeutic techniques and selections of scripts in working with a variety of problems. In case histories, names have been changed and minor historical information has been altered to protect the identity of the client. Scripts have been developed over the years and from many different sources. If I know the basic source of the script, I will give credit by indicating that the script is "adapted from . . ."

INTRODUCTION

There are many definitions of hypnosis but some common threads run through most of these definitions. These common threads indicate that hypnosis is (1) an altered state of awareness with, (2) focused concentration, (3) by-passing of the critical factor of the conscious mind, (4) conscious and subconscious communication, and (5) higher susceptibility to suggestion.

Though I may not be able to give you a detailed definition of hypnosis, I can tell you that it works. A few years ago, my son and I had just seen a world famous magician do one of his baffling tricks on television. My son turned to me and said, "How did he do that?" I replied, "Scott, I don't have the faintest idea." When we witness something that we do not understand or can not explain, we ask, "How did he do that?" When we see a good Hypnotherapist at work, we sometimes ask, "How did he do that?" We want to understand. We want to know. Sometimes we just have to learn the techniques and use them even when we can't answer the question "How did he do that?"

Some professional counselors, ministers, and medical doctors say they do not use hypnosis because they do not know how it works. They miss a valuable tool for counseling and self-help. If someone offered you a television set, would you say, "Oh no, I can't accept it because I don't know how it works." You don't have to know how a TV works to enjoy its benefits.

In addition to having many definitions, there are many approaches to hypnotherapy. You have read of or attended seminars about such clinical uses of hypnotherapy as Analytical Hypnotherapy, Ericksonion Hypnotherapy, Client-Centered Hypnotherapy, Alchemical Hypnotherapy, Power Hypnotherapy, Conflict Therapy Hypnotherapy, Hypno-Analysis, Hypno-Think, Time-Line Therapy, Parts Therapy, Clinical Hypnotherapy, and others that I failed to mention. I admit that I have learned much from each of these techniques and some of each will be found in how I use hypnotherapy.

The foundation for my work in hypnotherapy is based upon what I refer to as the human trinity, thus *Human Trinity Hypnotherapy.* Whether you are a Christian or not, you would probably know what I meant if I referred to the Holy Trinity: God the Father, the Son, and the Holy Spirit. I also believe in the human trinity. Each of us is a trinity within himself or herself. I am a trinity, you are a trinity. We are made up of body, mind, and spirit. We are physical, emotional and spiritual beings.

These three aspects of our being are so different and yet so integrated that one part of the human trinity can not be affected without having some effect on the other two. If you have a physical problem, it affects you emotionally and spiritually. That does not mean that if you are sick physically, you are also sick emotionally and spiritually, but that they are affected. A person with an illness may grow emotionally and spiritually as a result of the illness. It may be for good or bad but all three are affected. If you have an emotional problem, it affects you physically and spiritually. If you have a spiritual problem, if affects you physically and emotionally.

To demonstrate the effect of the emotional and spiritual on the physical, have a friend stand in front of you with his/her dominate arm outstretched at shoulder level. Push down on the arm and have the person resist. Have the person think a happy thought and resist. Push down and feel the resistance. Now ask the person to let the happy thought go and replace it with a sad thought. As the person thinks of a sad thought, push down. You will discover that the resistance is weakened. The difference between the happy thought and the sad thought resistance is obvious. If a sad or negative thought can cause one to lose power in his arm, what happens if one goes day after day, week after week, month after month thinking negative thoughts? The logical conclusion is that how one thinks and feels emotional or spiritual has an effect on one's body for good or bad.

In an article in the *Journal of the American Board of Hypnotherapy*, O. Carl Simonton states that the power of the mind goes far beyond what he first imagined. In addition, he believes that beyond the body and mind, there is another aspect of healing that needs to be addressed—the spiritual aspect.

The dictionary defines spirit as the life principle, especially in humans, and the feeling and motivation part of our lives. Working with spirit means enhancing our connection with the life principle. It means asking questions about why we're here on this planet, and about our unique purpose in life.

Simonton's work with patients has demonstrated that health involves body, mind, and spirit. And while the mind alone can be used to influence the physical state, it is used most effectively when it is aware of spirit. Spirit gives us resources that can't be reached through traditional psychological approaches. It opens us to healing forces that go far beyond our current understanding of our own limits. Simonton concludes, "We can learn to bring that power into our own lives."

According to an old legend, a spider let itself down from the peek of a barn by a silken thread until it reached a cross beam. There the spider spun an elaborate web, supported by the original thread. So interested did the spider become in what it had accomplished . . . and so proud . . . that it cut the supporting thread because there seemed to be not further need of it. The entire web collapsed, the spider was caught in its own web and died. We come into this world from the hand of God and on that hand, we are still dependent for the essential needs of life. No doubt God is pleased when we find new wonders in God's creation, but many have become so fascinated with the creation that they have forgotten the creator. We need to develop that spiritual side of our nature in order to reach our potential and live life more abundantly.

Accepting the theory of the human trinity, one understands that life is more than just being alive mentally and physically. To illustrate this, I would like to share two favorite stores which I use often. If you are aware that these stories were in my book, *Human Trinity Hypnotherapy,* remember that repetition is a learning tool in and out of hypnosis.

An airplane does not cease to be an airplane when it sits in the hanger or takes off along the runway, but its true nature becomes apparent only when it is airborne. Similarly, a person is a human being even when he or she is functioning only on the physical and psychological planes, but one shows his essential humanness when he rises to the spiritual dimension.

A man asked his three daughters how much they loved him. The oldest of them replied that she loved him more than all the gold and silver in the world. The father was noticeably pleased with her answer and gave her a big hug. The second daughter responded, "I love you more than the most valuable jewels in the world." He was pleased with her response and so he gave her a big hug. The third and youngest said, "I love you better than salt." The man was not especially elated with her remark and dismissed it lightly as an indication of her immaturity. Nevertheless, he gave her a hug. His wife, their mother, overhearing the conversation, left salt out of her husband's next meal. As he ate, he was thus confronted with the deep meaning of his youngest daughter's remark. She was saying that he was the flavoring and spice of her life. Developing the spiritual aspect is to life what salt is to food. The spiritual dimension gives flavor and seasoning to life. When one is functioning on all levels (physical, emotional and spiritual), life is more productive and more healthy.

Regardless of what you call your particular activity in hypnotherapy, we are all frog kissers. You may ask, "What is a frog kisser?" "Well did you ever feel like a frog?" You may respond, "How should I know what a frog feels like?" Maxie Dunnan in his book, *Barefoot Days of The Soul* ((1975) Word Books. Waco, Texas), tells us that frogs feel slow, low, puffy, drooped and pooped. The frog feeling comes when a person wants to be intelligent, but feels dumb, when he wants to share, but is selfish, when he wants to do right, but does wrong, when he wants to change, but does not, when he wants to care but is indifferent, when he wants to be accepted, but fells rejected, when he wants to stop a habit, but keeps on doing it. Yes, at one time or another, each of us have found ourselves on a lily pad, floating down the great river of life, disgusted but too froggish to budge.

Do you remember the fairy tale about a frog? Once upon a time there was a frog but he wasn't really frog. He was a prince who looked and felt like a frog. A wicked witch had cast a spell on him. Only the kiss of a beautiful young maiden could save him, but since when do cute girls go around kissing frogs? So there he sat—an unkissed prince in frog form. Though the situation seemed to be hopeless, miracles do happen. One day a beautiful young woman grabbed him up and gave him a big kiss right on his lips. Crash—boom—zap! There he was kissed—a frog before, a prince after.

As Hypnotherapist, our calling is to symbolically kiss frogs. Kissing frogs not with our lips but listening to them and then by the use of suggestion, imagery and healing stories to help people make changes in their life so they can become a prince or a princess.

The most beneficial seminars that I have attended and hypnotherapy books that I have read have been those that deal not only with theory but how theory is put into therapy. I admit that I am a believer in the use of scripts but only when information from the client is integrated into the script. I use scripts like a swimmer uses a diving board at a swimming pool. The diving board is the taking off place, but the real therapy is getting into the water. So get into the water and kiss some frogs.

Section One
Contributions to Human Trinity Hypnotherapy

Though I had only one quote from Alfred Adler and two from Viktor Frankl in my book *Human Trinity Hypnotherapy,* they have had a profound influence in my life and therapy. In 1972 and 1973, I completed four quarters of Clinical Pastoral Education C.P.E. at Walter Reed Army Medical Center in Washington, D.C. When I went there, I was a very outgoing person but inside, I felt inferior. When someone gave me a compliment, I would smile and say, "Thank you," but inside I would discount the compliment.

During the second quarter of C.P.E., our supervisor, Chaplain Ray Stephens, assigned each student two pioneer psychologists and asked that we present a class on each. I was assigned Alfred Adler and Viktor Frankl. As I prepared for these two classes, I began to notice a change in how I felt about myself. I recognized my inferiority feelings could be overcome (Adler) and that I could have meaning and purpose in my life (Frankl). As a result of those two classes, I went from low man on the totem pole to a class leader. The transformation I experienced (physically, emotionally and spiritually) could be compared to a conversion experience.

Adler, Frankl, and others have contributed to my understanding of human personality and how I relate to an individual in the therapeutic situation. With that acknowledgement, I began this section with a salute to some individuals outside of the field of hypnotherapy who have contributed to my development of *Human Trinity Hypnotherapy* (Alfred Adler, Viktor Frankl, Maxwell Maltz, John Powell, and the Bible).

Chapter One
Alfred Adler's Contributions

Thyra Boldsen once wrote of Adler that he was real, whether he was joking or serious, whether in private discussion or in lectures, his real personality always seemed to say, "Life is holy, have reverence for life, everything which happens is important."

In 1870, Alfred Adler was born in a suburb of Vienna. He was the second of six children. In his youth, Adler suffered from rickets and could not walk until he was four. He once said, "For me any sort of movement was a strain and effort." A short time after he was able to walk, he developed pneumonia. Because of his clumsiness, he had several accidents which caused him embarrassment and pain. These early experiences with illnesses and accidents probably accounts for his theory of organ inferiority and finally of the inferiority feelings. Due to his many contacts with doctors as a child, Adler decided that he wanted to grow up to be a doctor. As a boy, he spent a lot of time reading the great classical writers, cultivating flowers and collecting pigeons.

In 1895, Adler received his medical degree from the University of Vienna Medical School. Because of his expressive speaking ability, his knack at quoting the Bible, Shakespeare and the Greek Tragedies, his understanding of the history of psychology and philosophy, he often was the center of attention in groups. Though Adler was never a Freudian Psychotherapist, Freud and Adler formed a close friendship until a split developed between the two.

In 1911, Adler felt that he could no longer be associated with Freud. He with nine of the thirty-five members of Freud's group withdrew and formed the Society of Individual Psychology. Adler considered each patient as a separate individual in whom memories differ greatly. It was his opinion that no life-experience can be viewed in isolation, but must always be regarded in relation to the total personality. He wrote, "Individuals do not form unconscious memories all around the same central motive; sexuality for instance. Every person has a different need, an inferiority for which he seeks compensation. The method of Individual Psychology begins and ends with the problem of inferiority." Adler considered Freud's focus on sex was overplayed and his theory of libido false. Adler felt that the sex instinct was important but not as important as the individuals sense of inferiority. Someone said that Adler destroyed love. Adler saw much more to love than sexuality. He dethroned sexuality and the pleasure principle in order to make place for love and happiness.

Adler developed a theory of personality based upon (1) inferiority feelings and compensation, (2) striving for superiority, (3) style of life, (4) social interest, (5) family constellation, (6) fictional finalist, (7) the creative self, (8) masculine protest, (9) the interpretation of dreams, and (10) theory of psychotherapy. I will discuss how some of these theories have affected me. Adler said, "We do not flatter ourselves, we have not explored the last and ultimate facts, nor have voiced the last truth. All we have attained cannot be more than part of the present knowledge and culture. And we are looking forward to those who are coming after us." If we, as hypnotherapists, would take that statement to heart, we would be much better off as a professional.

Though Adler would use terms like physical, psychic, and soul, he felt there was a unity of body, mind, and spirit. The psychic attitude affects the physical and the physical affects the psychic. The soul has an affect upon and is affected by the physical and psychic.

According to Alder, each individual has a weak area in his/her body (organ inferiority) which tends to be the area where illness occurs—such as the stomach, head, heart, back, lungs, etc. Adler states that to some degree every emotion finds some expression in the body. The emotion will be seen in some visible form such as in the person's posture. The emotion may be seen in the face or trembling of a person's leg, changes can also take place in the organs of the body and the circulation of the blood. If we examine more closely, we shall find that every part of the body is involved in an emotional expression, and that the physical expressions are the consequences of the action of the mind upon the body.

Organ inferiority may lead one to excel in a certain area of life. Adler described the process of compensation for physical disabilities or limitations. The behavior may be satisfactory or unsatisfactory depending on the attitude the person takes toward his defects. Favorite examples of a good outcome are Demosthenes, who became a great speaker in compensation for an early defect in speech; Annette Killerson, who became a champion swimmer despite her body weakness, and limping Nurmi, who became a famous runner. Others with similar problems who did not compensate by excelling have sometimes used their defect as an excuse to reserve the fantasy that they would have gained prestige had they not had the defect. Adler wrote, "One may easily detect in every instance from observation of the child and from abnormalities of the adult that the possession of definitely inferior organs is reflected upon the psyche; and in such a way as to lower self-esteem and to raise the child's psychological uncertainty. It is just out of this lowered self-esteem that there arises the struggle for self-assertion which assumes forms much more intense than one would expect."

An illustration of a physical problem used as an excuse is discussed in *Human Trinity Hypnotherapy* (p. 19). A very prominent man was stricken with a stroke. He was the son of a famous man and had followed his father in their business. Though he was successful, he could not accept that fact. In comparison to his father, he felt like a failure. Following the stroke, he now had an excuse for his inability to reach the heights that his father had attained. He could now say, "If I had not suffered this damn stroke, I would have been as famous as my father."

From his understanding of organ inferiority, Adler began to see each individual as having a feeling of inferiority. Adler wrote, "To be a human being means to feel oneself inferior." The child comes into the world as a helpless little creature surrounded by powerful adults. A child is motivated by his feeling of inferiority to strive for greater things. When he has reached one level of development, he begins to feel inferior once more and the striving for something better begins again which is the driving force of mankind.

Every person has these feelings of inferiority whether or not he will or can admit it. Adler wrote, "Since the feeling of inferiority is regarded as a sign of weakness and as something shameful, there is naturally a strong tendency to conceal it. Indeed, the effort of concealment may be so great that the person himself ceases to be aware of his inferiority as such, being wholly preoccupied with the consequences of the feeling and with all the objective details that subserves its concealment. So efficiently may an individual train his whole mentality for the task that the entire current of his psychic life flowing ceaselessly from below to above, that is, from feelings of inferiority to that of superiority, occurs automatically and escapes his notice. It is not surprising, therefore, that we often receive a negative reply when we ask a person whether he has a feeling of inferiority. It is better not to press the point, but to observe his psychological movements, in which the attitude and individual goal can always be discerned."

Both the healthy individual and the neurotic individual copes with their feelings of inferiority by compensatory action through gaining power to overcome the sense of weakness. Their aggressive reaction often leads to considerable success in terms of recognized achievement in some area of life; some accomplishment of power over others. The neurotic compensates by denial or retreat. Such denial or retreat may take the form of fantasies, psychosomatic illness, projection, denial of reality, and other defense mechanisms.

These feelings of inferiority activates a person to strive upward so that normal feelings of inferiority impels the human being to solve his problems successfully, whereas the inferiority complex impedes or prevents him from doing so. It should be noted that inferiority feelings are different from inferiority complex.

The healthy individual will strive to overcome her inferiority through involvement with society. She is concerned about the welfare of others as well as herself. She develops a good feeling of self-worth and self-assurance. On other hand, some are more concerned with selfishness than with social interest. She may express this selfishness in the need to dominate, to refuse to cooperate, wanting to take and not to give. From these unhealthy responses, the person develops an inferiority complex or a superiority complex. A superiority complex is a cover up for an inferiority complex. They are different sides of the same coin. The person with a superiority complex has hidden doubts about her abilities.

Adler noted that all our thinking is goal-directed and forms a unified style of life. Each person has a specific goal which is all his own and makes him different from any one other person. As he follows that goal, he adopts early in life to specific technique for attaining that goal.

Adler describes four basic life styles: (1) The well-adjusted individual who does not strive for personal superiority, but seeks to solve his problems in ways that are useful to others as well as himself. (2) The type who wants to prove his personal superiority by ruling others. (3) The type who wants to get everything through others without any effort or struggle on his own. (4) The type who avoids every decision. Adler believed that an almost radical change in character and behavior will take place when the individual adopts new goals. The way to help a person with any negative responsive life style is to help that person move from reacting wrongly to life by changing his way of viewing life. People can change, the past can be released so that the individual is free to be happy in the present and the future.

Adler's Fictional Finalist is an interesting concept for the hypnotherapist. Adler was greatly influenced by Hans Voikinger's *Psychology Of The "As If"*. People act as much from the "as if" as from reality. One of my understandings of the subconscious mind is that whatever the subconscious mind accepts as true, it acts "as if" it were true whether it is or not.

The four phases of Adlerian counseling are: (1) the relationship, (2) the investigation of dynamics, (3) interpretation of the client, and (4) reorientation. Adler departed from Freud's method of having the client recline on a couch while the therapist sits behind. Adler preferred to face the client so he could see the client's responses and body movement. He wanted to engage in free discussion with the client. The relationship with the client which the Adlerian seeks to establish is one of friendliness and cooperation.

The investigation aspect explores the current life situation as it is viewed by the client to include his complaints, problems and symptoms. The client's early life and position in the family constellation are discussed. Adler believed that the order of birth is an important determiner of personality. The first born is given a great deal of attention until the second child is born and the first is dethroned. The dethroning experience may affect the child in a number of ways such as protecting himself from reversals, hatred for the second child, conservatism, insecurity, or it may cause him to develop a striving to protect others and be a helper.

The second child is in a different situation for he shares attention from the beginning which may cause him to be more cooperative or competitive. He may strive to catch and surpass the older child. All other children are dethroned but never the youngest, who is often spoiled. He may strive to overcome all the others. Adler used the Biblical story of Joseph who was the favorite of his father and the smartest of all his other children to illustrate that striving. It is true that Joseph had a younger brother, but he was 17 years younger than Joseph.

Some favorite questions of Adler were, "And why do you feel like that? What purpose does your illness serve? What do you think is the reason for your reacting that way?" The interpretation puts an emphasis on the goal and life style of the client. The mirror technique is used whereby the individual looks at himself.

During the reorientation stage, the client is encouraged to drop the old style of life and take up another. The new life style will be such as to help him deal with the realities of life and receive satisfaction from living.

Adler compares the client with a person who is caught in a dark room and cannot find an exit. The therapist helps the client illuminate the room so that she can find a way out to a new way of dealing with the problem. Adler wrote, "Every individual represents both a unity of personality and the individual who fashions that unity. The individual is thus both the picture and the artist." Therefore if one can change his concept of himself, he can change the picture he is painting.

Adler had very little to say about hypnosis, but what little he did say indicated that he did not understand the clinical possibilities of hypnosis. He recognized that no one could be hypnotized against his will, but felt that the individual who allowed himself to be hypnotized place himself under the power of the hypnotist.

(1) Beverly's Case History

Beverly was in the hospital for a skin graft to cover a large scar on her left leg. She was very self conscious about the scar and felt that people stared at her leg. I was consulted to work with her for pain management and self-esteem. Beverly was an illegitimate child who was raised by her grandparents. Though she knew who her mother was, she considered her like a sister and called her grandmother "mother." Her grandparents were strict—they set limits and always wanted to know where she was or had been. Beverly felt their limits were an indication of their love for her. She said "I had the hurts and accidents of childhood, but my grandparents were always there to show me love."

Beverly had a very close friend, Kay, who was "like a sister." It was Kay who told her about sex and to whom she went to for sexual advice. Beverly had not been given any instructions concerning menstruation, so she was very frightened when she first started at age 11. Kay told her what was happening and then everything was all right.

As she began to develop sexually, she felt good because she wanted to catch up with Kay who was two years her senior. "She was like a sister and I wanted to keep up with her. I felt really grown up. It was exciting. I thought, 'Great, now I am catching up with Kay; everyone will be proud of me'." This is in line with Adler's view that the younger child wants to catch up with the older child.

Following high school, Beverly joined the army and spent four years on active duty. Shortly after she was released from the army she had an accident on a bicycle which was the cause of the large scar on her leg.

To help her cope with pain and increase her self-esteem, I used several techniques and scripts while counseling Beverly. Beverly was a visual person with a slight dominance for indirect suggestibility.

(2) Setting Sun for Tranquility and Healing

See (If person was not visual, I would use "imagine") yourself sitting on a tropical beach at sunset. Notice the bright sun as it descends on the far horizon. See the colors begin to change from orange to crimson, and then to a deep, red-orange. Notice that as the sun approaches the water, there actually seems to be two suns, one in the sky and the other in the water. See the sun gradually sink into the ocean. See the colors change from red to purple and then to blue. Notice the magical stillness that pervades everything just at sunset when the ocean is as smooth as glass. Enjoy the delicious feeling of tranquility . . .

And perhaps you can begin to remember that God created within you an inner, central core of existence, that place deep within the central part of your mind and a place of inner healing power and life force. And remembering that from the very beginning of existence, the mind and body have known how to heal themselves. The body knows how to heal the cuts and wounds and injuries, how to generate new cells and new tissue whenever needed. And the body knows equally well how to regulate its only healthy functioning; regulating heart rate and breathing, and body temperature and blood pressure: all effortlessly, subconsciously, automatically maintained at healthy levels . . .

The subconscious mind knows how to maintain its own healthy blood chemistry, and maintain the necessary hormonal and chemical components for a healthy functioning mind and body. The subconscious mind knows how to maintain and regulate the proper level of potassium, of endorphins, all the necessary hormonal and chemical components that allow for an active, alert mind and body; but without over stimulation . . .

And in similar fashion, the subconscious mind is maintaining an immune system effortlessly, automatically, and warding off invading organisms before they have a chance to gain a foothold. Building resistance, maintaining resistance, building antibodies, the white blood cells surrounding the invading viruses or bacteria, like fearless knights on beautiful horses. And the subconscious mind knows how to regulate its metabolic system; the metabolism being designed to help us stabilize our bodies at a normal, moderate, healthy level. And in every way, mind, spirit and body work for health; healing maintenance of healthy functioning, and somehow recognize these inner resources—the strength, the growth, the healing, the life force, making everything easier. Day by day in every way, you are getting better and better, healthier and healthier.

(3) Building Self-Confidence and Self-Esteem

You are feeling relaxed and peaceful. As you are relaxed and peaceful, you feel good about yourself. This good feeling is an experience you enjoy. You like the way you look, the way you feel. You realize that you can be more efficient and effective.

You feel good—now, you feel safe—now, you feel healthy—now. You enjoy life—now. Your self-esteem, self-confidence, self-acceptance is increasing with each breath you take. Everyday you become emotionally calmer, stabler, settled.

You realize that you are becoming the person you want to be. Hold this good image of yourself and allow it to sink into your subconscious, so that you have a model to work with. St. Paul said, "Whatsoever a person sows, that shall he reap." If a farmer goes to his field and sows corn seeds, that is what will grow. Now the farmer will need to keep the weeds out of his field by keeping the field clean of weeds. If you sow seeds of self-confidence, your self-confidence will grow. You need to keep out negative attitudes and doubts about yourself so that your self-confidence continues to increase.

You are learning to love yourself. You like yourself. You are realizing that loving yourself is not selfishness. Selfishness is the opposite of self love. A selfish person does not love herself and lacks a feeling of self-worth. As you begin to love yourself, you see your worth as a person and you can better relate to and love others. Perhaps that is what Jesus meant by "love your neighbor as yourself." As you love yourself, you can conquer destructive forces of negative thinking, worry, resentment, fear, and anxiety.

Each day you keep improving physically, emotionally, mentally, and spiritually. You realize that you are good. You have a greater sense of personal well-being and you feel more secure. Your self-confidence, self-acceptance and self-esteem grows stronger everyday in every way. Repeat several times, "I am self-confident and day by day in every way my confidence is increasing."

You have outstanding capability. You have within you more mental and creative power than you ever thought possible. As you begin to see yourself as a person of worth, your motivation is increasing, your self-confidence is increasing. Day by day, you are getting better and better, healthier and healthier, happier and happier. Are you becoming more self-confident because I suggest it or because you are learning to be self-confident? You progressively feel better about yourself as your self-esteem increases everyday. It is a cycle of progress . . .

Beverly now feels good about herself and has a life style that is undergirded with social interest. As she has a concern for others as well as herself, I feel that she will have a very satisfying life. Beverly is basically a well adjusted person who can function well in society.

(4) Alfred Adler's Bibliography

Adler, A. (1969). *Individual Psychology.* Littlefield and Adams. Totowa, N.J.

Adler, A. (1964). *Problems of Neurosis.* Harper Tourchbook. N.Y.

Adler, A. (1964). *Social Interest.* Capricorn Book. N.Y.

Adler, A. (1973). *Superiority and Social Interest.* Viking Compass Book. N.Y.

Adler, A. (1954). *Understanding Human Nature.* Faucet. Greenwich, CT

Ansbacher, H. and R. (1956). *The Individual Psychology of Alfred Adler.* Basic Book. N.Y.

Dreikus R. (1953). *Fundamentals of Adlerian Psychology.* Alfred Adler Institute. Chicago, Ill.

Mosak, H. (1973). *Alfred Adler: His Influence on Psychology Today.* Noyer Press. Park Ridge, N.J.

Orgler, B. (1956). *Alfred Adler: The Man And His Work.* A Mentor Book, N.Y.

Chapter Two

Viktor Frankl's Contributions

Viktor Frankl was one time Professor of Psychiatry at the University of Vienna Medical School and later taught at a number of schools in the United States. Frankl's first book in English was *Man's Search for Meaning* which he wrote while in a Nazi prison during World War II. He spent three years in various Nazi prison camps and experienced incredible suffering and degradation, but through those experiences further developed his theory of Logotherapy. Dr. Frankl's "Logotherapy" has had a profound influence on my life and therapy.

Frankl calls his therapy "Logotherapy." "Logos" is the Greek word for "meaning." Logotherapy focuses on the meaning of human existence as well as man's search for meaning. According to Frankl, the striving to find meaning in one's life is the primary motivational force in man. In using the term "man," Frankl is referring to the "human race:" male and female. Frankl sees man as a whole which includes body, mind, and spirit. All three are interwoven together so that each affects the other. He uses the example of a glass. To look at the glass from one view it looks like a glass; from another direction, a circle; and to see the shadow is to view another shape.

Frankl not only recognized man's spirit, but actually starts from it. It must be kept in mind that for Frankl "spiritual" does not have a religious connotation, but refers to the specific human dimension. I would like to point out that Frankl was very friendly toward religion and did not hesitate to use it if his patients were inclined toward religion.

Though logotherapy is not concerned with helping a person experience a belief in God, time and time again that is just what occurred. The fact that a person's faith is renewed is based upon the fundamental assumption of logotherapy which form a chain of interconnected links: (1) freedom of will, (2) will to meaning, and (3) meaning to life.

Frankl says that there are two classes of people who maintain that man's will is not free: schizophrenic patients and deterministic philosophers, psychologists, theologians, and others who hold a deterministic view of man. Frankl believed that humans determine themselves whether to give in to conditions or stand up to them. People are ultimately self-determining. People have the capacity to rise above conditions and transcend them. Human freedom must be recognized, or else religion is a delusion and education an illusion. Frankl admits that our freedom is freedom within limits. We are not free from conditions, but we always remain free to take a stand toward those conditions. We always retain the freedom to choose our attitude toward them. I integrate this idea of freedom to choose our attitude toward condition in most of my counseling.

Humans are ultimately self-determining. What one becomes within limit of endowment and environment, he has made for himself. Frankl wrote, "In the concentration camp, for example, in this living laboratory and on this testing ground, we watched and witnessed some of our comrades behave like swine while others behaved like saints. Man has both potentialities within himself; which one is actualized depends on decisions but not on conditions. Our generation is realistic, for we have come to know man as he really is. After all, man is that being who invented the gas chambers of Auschwitz, and he is also that being who entered those gas chambers upright, with the Lord's Prayer or the Shema Yisrael on his lips."

The will to meaning for Frankl was the basic striving for humans to find fulfillment, meaning, and purpose. Man is reaching out to the world, a world which is replete with other beings to encounter and meanings to fulfill. Such a view is profoundly opposite to those motivational theories which are based on the homeostasis principles. According to those who accept the homeostasis principle, man is basically concerned with maintaining or restoring an inner equilibrium tension and for experiencing the goal of gratification of drives and satisfaction of needs.

It was Frankl's contention that the pleasure principle is self-defeating. The more one aims at a pleasure, the more his aim is missed. The very "pursuit of happiness" is what thwarts it. Pleasure is missed when it is the goal and attained when it is the side effect of attaining a goal. Hypnotherapists call this the Law of Reversed Effect: "The harder you try . . . the more difficult it becomes."

I am reminded that in the Museum of the State House of Mississippi there is an old rusty breastplate and sword. They are relics of the first expedition of the Spanish to Florida and the lands to the west. They came in search of gold, but found only monotonous stretches of sand, dense forest, poisonous snakes, insects, wild beasts, and hostile people. They were at times discouraged, disheartened, and ready to quit. On other occasions, they were feverish with hope from the report that gold was just around the bend, just over the hill, or just across the river. It seemed the further they went in search of gold, the further from gold they got. Is not this a parable of life?

People seek the gold mine of meaning and happiness. All of us are investing our life in one gold mine or another. The drunkard with his bottle; the dope abuser with his pills, smokes, needles; the student at her desk; the woman with her work; the man at his task—all in quest of the gold mine of happiness. This quest was given a place in our American Declaration of Independence. Our founding fathers stated that we have certain rights, among them "the right to life, liberty, and the pursuit of happiness." We crave happiness, we demand it as a right, we seek it with all our power, yet many of us are missing all too much of it.

We have been missing happiness because we have been so set, so intense, so concentrated on finding happiness that we were unable to recognize that happiness does not come by searching for it, but because of something else. The pursuit of happiness turns out to be an impossible search. Happiness is the by-product of a meaningful life.

To live a meaningless life is to believe that there is motion without purpose, activity without a goal, pain without a reason. Don Heiges tells of a group of laborers who blasted through asphalt and concrete streets with air hammers and then dug to a depth five feet. After they finished, the boss would inspect the hole and say to the laborers, "OK, you can fill it up now." This seemingly pointless routine went on all morning long and the workers were becoming weary. At noon, the laborers came to the foreman and announced, "We quit, pay us and we will leave." The foreman was astonished by their attitude and so asked whether the work was too hard or the pay too low. One of the workers, acting as spokesman said, "The pay's OK and the work can be done, but we quit because no one is going to make a fool of us—digging holes and filling them up." Now knowing the cause of their unrest, the foreman explained that records had been lost and they were trying to locate the water pipes. With that explanation, the men went back to work. They could now see some meaning to their digging holes and filling them up again.

So often our lives seem to be without meaning, but unlike those workers, we just go on digging holes and filling them up. Many believe that their life has no purpose, no challenge. They feel it makes no difference what they do or do not do, and that life is overpowering. They come to feel that they are hopelessly trapped by circumstances beyond their control, that they are being defected by life, that life is a rat race, a treadmill, and that there is no meaning in their lives. This meaninglessness becomes a vacuum in one's soul. Some try to fill that vacuum by extra work, by parties, by games, by dope, by alcohol, by sex, by defiance of authority, speedy cars, committee work, watching television, over-eating, and indulgence in various other activities.

Man is pushed by his drives and pulled by meaning. This implies that it is always up to the individual to decide whether or not he wishes to fulfill the later. Meaning and fulfillment always implies decision-making; thus, a will to meaning rather than a drive to meaning. The meaning of life differs from person to person, from day today, and from hour to hour. What matters is not the meaning of life in general but rather the specific meaning of a person's life at given moment. Everyone has his own specific vocation or mission in life. Everyone must carry out a concrete assignment that demands this fulfillment. Everyone's task is unique as is his specific opportunity to implement it. It is the individual's responsibility to come to an understanding of the meaning of his life.

The therapist's role consists in widening and broadening the visual field of the client so that the spectrum of meaning and values become conscious and visible to them. Meaning of life may change, but it never ceases to be. We can discover meaning through creative values, experience values and attitudinal values. Meaning can come through what we give to life (creative values), by what we take from the world: listening to music, reading, etc. (experience values), and through the stand we take toward a situation we can no longer change such as the death of a loved one (attitudinal values). As long as one remains conscious, he is under obligation to realize values, even if it is only attitudinal values. Frankl does not claim to have an answer for the individual's meaning of life. Meaning must be found but it cannot be given. Logotherapy is an optimistic approach to life, for it teaches that there are no tragic or negative aspects which cannot, by the stand one takes to them, be translated into positive accomplishments.

The therapist is faced with the seemingly impossible twofold task of considering the uniqueness of each person, as well as the uniqueness of life situations with which each person has to cope. The choice of an appropriate therapy to be used depends on the individual client and your relationship with the client. The relationship between two persons seems to be the most significant aspect of the therapeutic process, a more important factor than any method or technique.

It is commonly observed that anxiety often produces precisely what the client fears. Frankl called this "anticipatory anxiety." For instance, in cases of insomnia, the client reports that they have been having trouble going to sleep at night. The fear of not going to sleep only adds to difficulty of trying to go to sleep. Many sexual problems (impotency, failure to experience orgasm) are intensified by anticipatory anxiety.

Frankl developed the technique of "paradoxical intention." For instance, when a phobia client is afraid that something will happen to them, the logotherapist encourages them to intent or wish for, even if only for a short time, precisely what they fear. Hypnotherapists call this method or a slight variation of it, "desensitization." I have used "paradoxical intention," with a lady who ate two bags of popcorn each night and wanted to stop. During the counseling session, I said to her, "Now, tonight just say to yourself: 'Well, I have been eating two bags of popcorn each night. Tonight, I am going to eat four bags of popcorn. If I can eat two bags of popcorn, I can surely eat four bags'." She begin to laugh and said, "That is ridiculous. I don't want four bags. Two bags are too much also. I can be satisfied with one or less." You may notice that there can be a touch of the ridiculous and humor in this approach. Paradoxical intention allows the client to develop a sense of detachment toward his problem by laughing at it.

This procedure is based upon the fact that problems are caused as much by the compulsion to avoid or fight them as any problem itself. To avoid or fight the problem focuses on the problem and results in the strengthening of the symptom. By exaggerating the problem, one may observe that the symptoms diminish and the client is no longer haunted by them (circle therapy).

There is meaning to life and it is unconditional meaning. Life has meaning and neither suffering nor dying can distract from it. Frankl wrote of an unconditional trust in the ultimate meaning and unconditional faith in the ultimate being, God. Habakkuk chanted his triumphant hymn: "Although the fig tree shall not blossom, neither shall fruit be in the vines, the labor of the olive tree shall fail, and the fields shall yield no meat; the flock shall be cut off from the fold, and there shall be no herd in the stalls, yet I will rejoice in the Lord, I will joy in the God of my salvation." (3:17-18) Frankl concludes his book, *The Will to Meaning,* with that Biblical quote and this statement, "May this be the lesson to learn from my book."

(1) Mr. Wilder's Case History

Mr. Wilder, a 70-year-old man, came to me because he could not get over the death of his wife. Since his wife's death about a year before, he felt he had no meaning and had lost the will to live. He worried about many things, much of which was beyond his control. He said, "I worry about everything from the state of the economy to my own personal safety. I have no reason to get up in the morning. I spend most of my time at home and some days, I do not even get dressed. I just spend the day in my PJ's. I still go to church, but that's about all I do."

I had three sessions with Mr. Wilder over a month's period. We worked together to help him accept his wife's death and to accept his worth as a person, to increase his self-confidence, and to find his meaning for his life. During his second session, I asked him, "What is it you can do to help others?" He thought for several minutes and responded, "In our church newsletter, I read about the need for volunteers at the hospital near my home. I would rather volunteer here at Methodist, but as you know I live across town. Maybe I could volunteer to work at the hospital near my home." I share with you some suggestions, imagery, and healing stories used with Mr. Wilder.

(2) The Goose in the Bottle

As you relax peacefully and comfortably, I would like to share with you a story. You have told me about how you worry about many things so may you allow this story to speak to you its message.

This is the story about a teacher who said to his students, "Let's make believe we've placed a goose egg into a bottle. The goose egg hatches and the goose begins to grow. Your assignment is to get the goose out of the bottle without breaking the bottle or injuring the goose."

One student thought and thought about this at great length. How could he get the goose out of the bottle without hurting the goose or breaking the bottle? Not being able to figure it out, he become so frustrated with the question that he could not sleep . . .

Finally he went to the teacher and said, "You must get the goose out of the bottle. The problem is driving me out of my mind. I can't figure it out." "Very well," said the teacher and continued, "bring me the bottle with the goose inside." It was only then that the student realized he had been struggling with a situation that did not actually exist . . . And so it is with some of the things you have been worrying about . . . They either do not exist or they are beyond your power to change . . . so let them go . . .

(3) Building Self-Confidence #2

The suggestions and instructions I'm telling you now are going into the storehouse of your subconscious mind and are progressively having a greater influence over you. Each day these suggestions keep becoming more effective, and they help you many different ways: physically, mentally, emotionally, and spiritually . . . The things that I say are influencing your thoughts, your feelings, and your actions in a positive and helpful way. Even after you come out of this hypnotic state these suggestions continue influencing you just as surely as they do while you are in the hypnotic state of relaxation . . .

You are pleased with the improvements in your life . . . The improvements are progressive. As each day passes, you continue improving more and you can be sure it is permanent and lasting . . . As I talk with you, you keep going into a deeper, more peaceful, more detached state . . . Everything I tell you becomes deeply reinforced in your mind, and your mind is causing it to work so you continue progressing in everything you do . . .

You can be more calm and relaxed during your daily life and that causes your mind to be more clear, more alert, and causes you to feel more refreshed. Your nerves continue to be more relaxed and steady. You are more composed, more tranquil and more at peace within . . . You automatically apply these principles of relaxation in all the activities of your daily life, and you can be peaceful and calm in every situation and circumstance in which you find yourself, whether you are alone or with others . . . This enables you to be more efficient in your life and it keeps increasing your self-confidence, your self-reliance, your self-acceptance and your self-esteem . . . You continue developing a more relaxed attitude, greater concentration, and you keep achieving more outstanding accomplishments: in your life you find ways to make your life more meaningful.

It's a cycle of progress that keeps growing stronger each day and causes you to continue advancing and enables you to become the successful person you are capable of being . . . Being more calm and relaxed enables you to think more clearly. You are able to focus your attention more readily, and it causes your memory to keep improving more each day.

You sleep much better when you desire to sleep. When you are ready to go to sleep, all of your muscles and nerves relax, and you easily go into a deep, peaceful state of sleep. When you awaken you feel rested and refreshed. Your mind is alert, and you are able to see and understand things in their true perspective, without magnifying them, or without letting them get out of proportion. You are healthier, stronger and have more energy from relaxing so peacefully as you sleep . . .

You are rapidly becoming the person you have always wanted to be: self-confident, self-sufficient, healthy, acceptable, capable and strong . . . You have many talents, many skills, and many abilities, therefore, you have many reasons to have confidence in yourself . . . You have the ability to experience a more joyful life. You enjoy life more each day. Your happiness keeps increasing and you are more optimistic . . . You feel more productive, more useful, more healthy, and experience more happiness . . .

(4) The Turning Point: Prince Andrew

Sometime ago, while visiting a book store, I saw a book, *The Turning Point.* Though I did not buy the book, it brought to mind that each of us face many turning points in our life. You are facing a turning point in your life today and you have the chance to make a positive change in your life.

There is an interesting incident in the book, *War and Peace* concerning Prince Andrew. The Prince has gone through a long period of grief and depression which had sapped his strength. He thought that his life had no meaning or purpose. As he traveled over his land in the winter, he passed an old oak tree which was bare of leaves and looked dead. He thought to himself, "I am like that tree."

It was not until the following spring that he traveled back across the same route where he had seen the old oak tree. Feeling as old, as tired, as meaningless, as depressed as ever, he came to the old oak tree. To his surprise, he noticed the oak tree had come to life. It had new leaves and new growth. The tree which he had identified himself was new, green, growing, and beautiful. It was a turning point for him as he realized new life, new meaning, new hope and new purpose was available for him as it was for the tree. New hope, new purpose, new meaning can be yours . . .

About a month after our last session, I talked to Mr. Wilder on the phone. He told me that he was working as a volunteer at the hospital near his home. He said, "Now I have a reason to get up in the morning and I am enjoying my life again."

(5) Viktor Frankl's Bibliography

Crumbaugh, J. (1973). *Everything to Gain: A Guide to Logotherapy.* Nelson-Hull, Chicago.

Frankl, V. (1957). *Doctor and the Soul.* Alfred Knox. N.Y.

Frankl, V. (1963). *Man's Search for Meaning.* Pocket Book. N.Y.

Frankl, V. (1967). *Psychotherapy and Existentialism.* Clarion Book. N.Y.

Frankl, V. (1970). *The Will to Meaning.* Plum Book. N.Y.

Stern, A. (1971). *The Search for Meaning.* Memphis State University. Memphis, TN.

Tweedie, Jr. R. (1961) *Logotherapy.* Baker Book House. Grand Rapids, MN.

Chapter Three

Maxwell Maltz's Contributions

Dr. Maxwell Maltz was a world famous plastic surgeon who discovered the incredible power of a person's self-image for good or bad. Over the years, he realized that people's real problems were not their outward physical appearance, but their inner self-image. Following this discovery, he wrote several books using his term, "Psycho-Cybernetics."

Over 20 years ago, I purchased a book titled, *Psycho-Cybernetics* by Dr. Maxwell Maltz. I admit that the title was not that impressive for I had no idea what "Psyco-Cybernetics" meant. I bought the book based upon its table of contents. Though the title was unimpressive, the content of that book and others by Dr. Maltz has had a profound influence on my life and therapy.

While preparing this chapter, I have reread five books and listened to eight audio tapes by Dr. Maltz. As I reread those books and listened to the tapes, I was surprised to notice how much Dr. Maltz had contributed to my understanding of the human condition.

In previous chapters, I wrote in regards to the effect Dr. Afred Adler and Viktor Frankl had on me. I found a lot of their ideas reflected by Dr. Maltz and reading his books just watered and fertilized the seeds planted by Adler and Frankl.

Many of Dr. Maltz's ideas regarding self-image, relaxation, imagery, forgiveness and mental programming entered my mind by osmosis so that when I talk or write, it seems like the ideas are all mine. Though I have only two footnotes of Dr. Maltz in my book, *Human Trinity Hypnotherapy,* those who read the book will see his spirit reflected through out that book.

As I read Dr. Maltz, I discovered that "Cybernetics" means "goal-seeker" and carries with it the image of a helmsman who steers a ship to port. "Psycho-Cybernetics" is the steering of one's mind to produce good thoughts and actions so that a person can achieve success, happiness and peace of mind. Areas I would like to highlight from Maxwell Maltz are self-image, relaxation, imagery, and forgiveness.

1. *SELF-IMAGE:* A person's self-image is a blueprint for his/her life and the person follows that blueprint (good or bad) until the blueprint (self-image) is changed. In one of the "Peanut" cartoons, Charlie Brown was standing next to a school house. Charlie said, "I hate being a nobody, I wish I

were a television star. If I were a TV star, I would not have to go to school." Next the school building spoke up, "I'd like to be the Sistine Chapel kid, but I'm not."

Charlie Brown's difficulty in thinking of himself as a somebody is a very real problem for a lot of people. Dr. Maltz points out that even some people who are considered successful are oppressed by a sense of personal insignificance. The inability to have a good self-image, to have a high opinion of one's self, to have a high level of self-worth is one of the greatest problems of our day. There are those who feel inferior and those who try to lord it over to others. The interesting thing is that they are both symptoms of a poor self-image. What is self-image? You can't see it, you can't touch it, you can't taste it; but nevertheless it is real. It is real as you can be. It is your blueprint for life. It is your inner picture of yourself. If is your opinion of yourself.

2. *RELAXATION:* The ability to change begins with the ability to relax. Dr. Maltz does not call this hypnosis but with the combination of relaxation and imagery, hypnosis is achieved. In the foreword to the latest edition of *Psycho Cybernetics,* hypnosis is explained as a part of the "normal operating process of the human brain and nervous system." When people are convinced that the hypnotists words are true statements, hypnotic subjects are able to easily produce remarkable phenomena. Dr. Maltz encourages the use of self-hypnosis to bring about change in the self-image.

   Dr. Maltz emphasizes the point that one cannot begin to properly develop new personality patterns until one becomes dehypnotized from negative input. The dehypnosis comes with hypnosis using different suggestions. Much hypnosis comes without a formal indication. It is not an exaggeration to say that we are more or less hypnotized whenever we uncritically accept an idea or statement as true. When a person uses self-hypnosis, a person can give himself audible or mental suggestions for the reprogramming of the mind. Progressive relaxation allows a person to reach a hypnotic state where she can change her self-image and thereby change her life.

3. *IMAGERY:* Imagination plays a far more important role in a person's life than most of us realize. A person acts and feels not according to what things are really like, but according to the image he holds in his mind about what they are like. The person has a certain metal image of himself, his world, and the people around him. The person lives and behaves based upon that image. By the use of "Creative Imagery," a person can change his self-image. A favorite technique of Dr. Maltz was "The theatres of your mind." Mental pictures of the way you want to be offers a person the opportunity to "practice" new traits and attitudes. Your subconscious mind cannot tell the difference between an actual experience and one that is vividly imagined. As a person recognizes their capabilities and imagines accomplishing what they want to happen, the subconscious mind begins to work out a way to make it happen. "The theatres of the mind" can be used whether you are a visual person or not. It works just as well with those who think mostly with inner voices, sounds, and feelings.

   One use of the mind is "step in-step out" techniques. This is helpful in releasing unpleasant memories. Remember an unpleasant memory, "step out" of the memory and watch yourself in it from the audience of your mental theatre. Make the screen as small and as far away as necessary to learn from it, without re-experiencing the unpleasant feelings. Repeat until the screen is so small you can not see it or feel it.

   Follow that with a series of pleasant memories on your mental movie screen. "Step in" to each memory, relieve each experience as if it were actually happening again. Allow yourself to feel the pleasant feeling fully. If you do this each day, your subconscious mind will begin to automatically draw you to a positive, pleasant experience and minimizes the negative effect of unpleasant experiences. A person can also use the "theatre of your mind" to picture himself doing what he wants to happen in his life and activities. These mental pictures become the person's reality and changes come to his life.

4. *FORGIVENESS:* One of the most destructive aspects of human life is the failure to forgive. Forgive others. Do it not only for their sake, but for your own. Dr. Maltz realized that people need psychological surgery. People need to remove

> emotional growths and scars. Forgiveness is used to remove emotional scars and guilt. A person should forgive even when the person who harmed him doesn't ask for nor desires forgiveness. A person needs to forgive in order to free himself from the power the other person has over him.
>
> Just as it is important to forgive others, it is equally important to forgive oneself. So often unresolved guilt (whether real or imaginary) creates a need to make amends, to make restitution, to suffer enough to pay back the wrong, to set things right by damage to self and thus to balance the account. Guilt, whether real or imagined must either be forgiven or punished. It is not God who punishes, but if a person does not feel forgiven, she will find a way to punish herself. The message is clear, forgive yourself and begin to live the more abundant life.

Dr. Maltz writes that God has offered us forgiveness, peace of mind, and happiness that comes with the forgiving of ourselves. The most adequate and realistic self-image of all is to conceive oneself that he is "made in the image of God." You cannot believe of yourself as made in the image of God, deeply and sincerely and not receive a source of strength and power. With this understanding, one is never too young or to old to change his self-image and start a new, more productive, more creative life. I close this discussion of Maxwell Maltz with a quote from the preface of his book, *The Magic Power of Self-Image Psychology.* "God brought us forth on the earth to live, not to stagnate. He meant us to be happy, to enjoy our lives. He meant us to relish every moment, to weave loving care on every day that we live—no matter how young or old we are."

(1) Ann's Case History

Ann is a 39-year-old female who came to me in hopes of finding relief from a panic disorder. She had trouble leaving her home and would leave home only with a few close friends. Even with friends, she felt uncomfortable. She had a fear of being alone. She said, "I need someone." Ann was very close to her mother, but felt forsaken by her father. "Dad was there but he was not available. He did not matter very much." Her father had abandoned her emotionally and she was afraid that her mother would also leave her.

She once said to me, "What is life without anxiety? If I don't have anxiety, I am dead." I asked her, "Can you replace happiness with anxiety and still be alive?" She replied, "I hope so."

(2) Theatre of the Mind

I saw Ann several times. In one session, I used Dr. Maltz's "theatre of the mind" which is a desensitization technique. I had her imagine a time when she was experiencing a panic attack. Now "step out" of that memory and watch yourself as on the screen from the audience of your mental theatre. Now make the screen small and as far away as necessary to experience the panic feeling being reduced. The further the picture goes, the smaller the picture becomes and the better you feel. Keep doing this until you are able to release all unpleasant feelings.

Now think of a very pleasant experience from your past on your mental movie screen. "Step into" that memory, relive that experience as if it were actually happening again. Allow yourself to feel the pleasant feeling fully. Do this over and over again replacing the happy memory with the panic memory until the happy memory clears away all other feelings.

(3) Waterfall for Cleansing

On another occasion, I used this script: Imagine that you are taking a walk in the woods. You are walking along a beautiful path. As you walk, you may experience a number of things. Possibly you are aware of the trees; some large, some small. It is a warm but comfortable summer day. Perhaps you feel a comfortable breeze . . . gently cooling your face and arms . . . maybe you can hear the rustling of the leaves and the crunch of the leaves, twigs, and grass beneath your feet. As you look up through the leaves of the trees, you see a sparkling of sunlight, and a beautiful blue sky with a few white clouds drifting by.

You come to an open area with a small pond. At one end of the pond is a beautiful waterfall. At the other end is a stream which runs as far as the eye can see. You sit down by the pond and enjoy the sounds of the waterfall, birds singing, and frogs croaking . . . as you sit there, you sense that there is something special about the waterfall. It seems to be inviting you to come over to it and indeed you do . . . you reach out and touch the water and the temperature is just right so you walk under the falls . . . you feel its cleansing flow and you realize that it is not only cleansing your body, but it also is cleansing your soul. You feel that any anger, bitterness, feeling of rejection, grief, guilt, panic, and all other negative emotions are being cleansed from your system.

You look down toward your feet and notice that the water coming from your body is a murky brown and it is flowing across the pond and down the stream at the other end. The more negative you release the murkier the water appears to be. As you feel these negative emotions being cleansed from your system, the water around your feet begins to clear, and you can see the murky brown water flowing further down the stream.

As the murky water flows down the stream, further and further away, you feel more and more comfortable, more at peace with yourself . . . it gives you a strong feeling of relief . . . you are feeling yourself being cleansed of all those negative feelings. The anger, bitterness, feelings of rejection, grief, guilt, abuse, panic, and all other negative emotions are being cleansed from your system . . . notice the feelings of comfort and peace increase as the murky brown water flows down the stream further and further away, you feel a sense of release and relief . . . you are getting rid of those problems . . .

The murky brown is flowing further and further away. It is now beyond your eye sight and you can breath deeper and exhale slowly a few times. Now really enjoy the freedom, the relief, the calmness, the peacefulness that flows through you and as it replaces the negative feelings. These feelings of comfort, serenity, and well-being remains with you even after you come out of the hypnotic state.

(4) I Love Me

There is something you have to do and it may not be easy but say out loud, "I love me." . . . "I love me." . . . This is not an egotistical attitude but it is the basis of your healing. The understanding of the value to loving yourself comes from the Old and New Testament. The writer of Leviticus 19:18, "You shall love your neighbor as yourself," and Jesus reaffirms the statement of Leviticus, "Love your neighbor as yourself" (Matthew 19:19).

Say, "I love me." . . . "I love me." . . . "I love me." . . . Now experience peace, feel good within yourself as you repeat, "I love me." . . . "I love me." . . . "I'm ok." . . . "I love others" . . . "I love others." . . . Jesus said, "The kingdom of God is within you." We are made in the image of God. There is a plaque which reads, "I'm me and I'm wonderful, because God don't make junk." The grammar may be incorrect, but the message is great. You are the handiwork of God and God don't make junk. You were created by God. God loves you. Love yourself and love that little child of your past. Give that little child the love she/he needs.

Let go of the past, the past is past. Perhaps you have heard the old saying, "The world is too much with us" . . . but in many cases the past is too much with us . . . Because the past contained an incident or several incidents in which you have conditioned yourselves wrongly . . . the past fouls up the present and makes the future seem dim. Therefore get rid of the past, not your memory of the past, but its impact upon you . . . The past is past. Let it go completely . . . now you can make it past by putting it in the past where it belongs. Now, do it right now, this very moment . . . the past is a cancelled cheque . . . the future is a promissory note . . . the present is cash . . . spend it wisely . . . say again, "I love me." . . . Let it vibrate in your mind and throughout your body, mind, and spirit. "I love me." . . . say it over and over again . . . You can handle the situation. You can overcome the problem. Life is worthwhile, life is meaningful, life is good. Love yourself, feel good about yourself, be calm within yourself, be at peace with yourself.

(5) Maxwell Maltz's Bibliography

Maltz, M. (1967). *Creative Living for Today.* Essondess Special Edition. N.Y.

Maltz, M. (1971). *The Magic Power of Self-Image Psychology.* Prentice-Hall Inc. Englewood, N.J.

Maltz, M. (1960). *Psycho-Cybernetic.* Pocket Book. N.Y.

Maltz, M. (1988). *Psycho-Cybernetic; (Workbook and 8 Audio Tapes).* Psycho-Cybernetic, Inc. Irvindal, CA.

Maltz, M. (1973). *Psycho-Cybernetic and Self Fulfillment.* Benton Book. N.Y.

Chapter Four
John Powell's Contributions

John Powell is a Catholic priest who has written a number of self-help books. He has taught Theology at Loyola University, Chicago, Catholic University of America, University of Notre Dome, and University of San Francisco. He has degrees in fields diverse as the Classics, English, Psychology, and Theology. John is a teacher, counselor, lecturer, and writer. I find that his thoughts, ideas and opinions have affected my thinking and understanding of life. I acknowledge his influence on my life and invite you to read his books for your own enhancement.

John Powell wrote an interesting book, *Why Am I Afraid to Tell You Who I Am?* When he told a friend about the book and mentioned the title, the friend asked, "Do you want an answer?" Powell responded, "Yes, of course." The friend said, "I am afraid to tell you who I am, because if I tell you who I am, you may not like me." To the extent that we experience hurt, anxiety, guilt, and inferiority feeling, we are tempted to build walls. These walls are our self-defense and we live behind them because we are afraid that we will be rejected if we are really known.

One of the important aspects of any counseling situation is rapport. Rapport is that accepting feeling on the part of the client to work with the therapist to help the client make meaningful changes in his life. It is the client's ability to trust the therapist in the counseling situation. In addition to skills and techniques, the hypnotherapist must establish rapport to be successful.

He quotes Dr. Paul Tournier, "No one can develop freely in the world without feeling understood by at least one person." As therapists we must be available to our clients so that they can open up and see us as that person that they can trust to hear them and keep on caring for them even when the dark secrets of their lives are discussed. Much of personal healing comes through a relationship with others who accept them unconditionally. An individual will either speak their feelings or act them out. Feelings are like steam that gathers inside a kettle. Steam is released or it builds up pressure and if the steam is keep inside the kettle, it will blow its top.

Without having someone to talk with, how is a person able to release the pressure that builds up inside without acting out the feelings. How will she/he be able to free themself from being a compulsive eater? How is the person who is angry inside going to release that anger in non-destructive ways without someone to talk with? How is someone who feels guilty going to experience forgiveness without someone to talk to? As a therapist, be loving, caring, and available so the person in need has someone to talk to in trust.

John Powell recognized that a good self-image is the most valuable psychological possession of a human being and a lack of self-worth is the most destructive aspect. Lack of self-worth brings depression, anger, antisocial behavior, physical sickness, addiction, feelings of meaninglessness, and a failure to live life to its fullest.

To have feelings of self-worth does not mean that a person has risen above his faults and emotional problems. It merely means that he refuses to be parked by them. The person who accepts and values himself as worthy is in the process of living a more abundant life. As he begins to love and appreciate himself, he finds that he loves and appreciates others more. John quotes Bertrand Russel, "A man cannot possibly be at peace with others until he has learned to be at peace with himself," and Jesus said, "Love your neighbor as yourself."

God is described as one who loves us unconditionally and desires the best for each of us. Jesus said, "I have come that you may have life and have it more abundantly." God's loving kindness is an unmerited gift and an irrevocable commitment. God said through the Prophet Isaiah, "Even if a mother should forget the child of her womb, I will never forget you" (Isaiah 49:15).

God does not punish us, but when we feel guilt, we find a way or ways to punish ourselves. When we separate ourselves from God and his love, all the changes take place in us, never in God. God loves us but we can refuse his love and the benefits his love brings to us. The story of the prodigal son (Luke 15:11-31) is a parable of God's unconditional love. When the father saw the wayward son returning home, he ran out to him and accepted him back as a son.

Powell understands the body, mind, spirit as the whole person. One part of that trinity cannot be affected without having an affect on the other two. He states that the American Academy of Psychosomatic Medicine has theorized that 92% of all physical illnesses are psychological induced. It would seem that many people, at least subconsciously, become sick because they have given up on the capacity to cope with life. If the mind and spirit can cause illness, a change in the mind and spirit can bring healing.

How do we change? To change, one must change one's thinking, the way one sees life, and vision of life. If a person has had a negative vision of life, she/he needs to begin by visualizing a better life, a happier life, a more meaningful life. "Vision therapy" is used with the belief that all changes in the quality of a person's life grows out of a change in his or her vision of reality. There can be no real and permanent change unless the negative, self-defeating vision is changed. The three requirements of "Vision therapy" are (1) find time for silence and solitude, (2) have an openness to face the questions of life, and (3) have a willingness to reverse one's interpretation of life. Socrates wrote, "The unreflected life isn't worth living."

In at last two of his books Powell quotes Viktor Frankl, and I would like to conclude this portion with a quote from *Man's Search For Meaning,* "A thought transfixed me: For the first time in my life, I saw the truth as it is set into song by many poets, proclaimed as the final wisdom by so many thinkers. The truth that love is the ultimate and highest goal to which man can aspire. Then I grasped the meaning of the greatest secret that human poetry and human thought and beliefs can import: The salvation of man is through love and in love."

(1) Ms. Jones' Case History

Ms. Jones, a 60-year-old woman, came to me for counseling with the statement that she could not get over the death of her son. Tom had died in an auto accident at the age of 21 some six months before Ms. Jones had called me. She felt depressed and wanted peace within. Whenever she tried to talk with someone about her grief, they would listen for a short time and then tell her it was time to leave it behind and get on with her life. Ms. Jones had a daughter who was 33 and a son 25, both live in the New Orleans area. She had been divorced for over 10 years and there was very little contact between the two since the divorce. Ms. Jones had several sessions over a four-month period.

(2) Cardinal Mercier: "We Will Rebuild"

While she was under hypnosis, I said to Ms. Jones, "I would like to tell you a story from World War II." Cardinal Mercier of Belgium was on a visit to Rome for a spiritual retreat. While he was in Rome, news reached him of the bombing of his home city. His Cathedral was in ruins, his library had been burned, but worst of all, many of his parishioners were dead.

In his grief, he cried, "Why all this sorrow? O Lord! My God, why has Thou forsaken us?" This was his gut reaction to the bad news he had received and the hurt of the loss of dear friends. As he began to cry, his face turned toward the cross. Though he continued to cry, he grew still. As he felt Christ come to him, he said with tears running down his face, "We will rebuild." He realized that God was still with him.

You have shared with me your faith in God so I am suggesting that you can this day experience the presence of God with you now. Allow God to help you rebuild your life. You can begin to imagine what you have to be thankful for. Can you name some of the things you have to be thankful for? A silence of about five minutes was ended when she said, "I am thankful for John and Mary (her two other children), their spouses and my four grandchildren. I have a good job and work with people who care about me. I have my church and God."

(3) Overcoming Depression

I concluded our last session with "Overcoming Depression," "Footprints in the Sand," and "Improving Self-Confidence." Now as you relax more deeply, let the cares of the world take care of themselves. Simply drift and float in your own pleasant thoughts. Let the sounds inside and outside this room contribute to your experience of relaxation and peace . . .

You came here Ms. Jones because you have had feelings of depression, meaningless, and lack of faith to met your grief. Yesterday you may have felt down and depressed. But I want you to know that today is new day; a new beginning . . . remember that saying, "Today is the beginning of the rest of your life." It's true . . . today is a very special and important day for you. Because you know that yesterday and all those sad feeling are a part of history . . . they are a part of your past. And you now choose to close the door on the past and leave behind any fears, doubts, and self-limitations. You keep those beautiful memories of Tom and the joy he brought to your life. You appreciate John and Mary and your grandchildren. You are thankful for your job, your church and God's love and presence with you . . .

(4) Footprints in the Sand

I want to tell you a story which you may have heard before, but which is a good story for you to consider today . . . one night a man had a dream. He dreamed that he was walking along the beach with God. As they looked back, he noticed two sets of footprints in the sand. One belonging to him and the other to God. Then across the sky flashed scenes of his life. When the last scene had flashed before him, he looked back at the footprints and noticed that many times along the path there was only one set of footprints in the sand. He also notice that this happened during the lowest and saddest times of his life. This really bothered him and he questioned God, "Lord, you said that once I decided to follow you, you would walk with me all the way, but I noticed that during the most troublesome times of life, there was only one set of footprints. I don't understand.

When I needed you most, you deserted me." God replied, "My precious, precious child, I love you and would never leave you. During your time of trial and suffering, when you see only one set of footprints, it was then that I carried you." God has carried you and continues to do so.

(5) Improving Self-Confidence

Ms. Jones, you accept and understand that today is new beginning of wonderful, exciting adventures in your life; a step toward the realization of your desire for inner peace and the attainment of your true and highest potentials . . .

As you continue to breath slowly and gently, you realize that you begin today to establish a new and solid foundation in your life. A foundation based on learning from past experience, of knowing where you want to go, and being confident that your choices are based on knowledge and wisdom . . .

You decide now to allow all the worries, fears, concerns, and problems of the past to just fade out of your life. You release them and let them go totally and completely. You know that God has a special purpose and plan for you. You are now open to that special purpose and plan. You put your life and trust in his hands. Remember Jesus said, "Ask and you shall receive, seek and you shall find, knock, and it shall be open to you" (Luke 11:9). So just as a child learns to walk one step at a time, you being today to pay close attention to all the good and wonderful things that are happening in your life . . .

When you face life positively, you realize that each and every experience you have leads you toward new understandings. So pay close attention to all the positive things happening around you. You are creating the exciting environment and space around you. You are now directing your own thinking. You're the programmer of your own destiny and master of your own life. You have the incredible freedom and power to chose to move positively in the directions you choose to move, and in doing so you realize that all your thoughts and actions are forming a remarkable image of yourself in your subconscious mind . . .

Be proud of who you are . . . believe in yourself . . . you have the right to exist just the way you choose to exist. Feel your new self-confidence. Let a warm swelling of pride emerge forth from within you. Have a respectful awe about yourself. Love yourself far more deeply now than you ever have before . . . feel it now . . . enjoy it now . . . take great delight in the wonderful gifts God has given you. Feel a deep sense of peace within you . . . feel your new happiness and the strength of your determination. Feel good as you experience a new beginning. Be thankful and let God's work continue to bloom in your life.

Ms. Jones has adjusted to life and feels that she has meaning and purpose for living. I see her from time to time in the community and she seems to be a happier and more contented person.

(6) John Powell's Bibliography

Powell, J. (1972). *A Reason to Live! A Reason to Die!* Argus Communication. Niles, Ill.

Powell, J. (1976). *Fully Human, Fully Alive.* Argus Communication. Niles, Ill.

Powell, J. (1974). *The Secret of Staying in Love.* Argus Communications. Niles, Ill.

Powell, J. (1978). *Unconditional Love.* Argus Communication. Niles, Ill.

Powell, J. (1969). *Why Am I Afraid to Love.* Argus Communication. Niles, Ill.

Chapter Five
The Bible's Contributions

Over the last four chapters, I have written about Alfred Adler, Viktor Frankl, Maxwell Maltz, and John Powell's contributions to Human Trinity Hypnotherapy. I could have also written about Maxie Dunnan, Keith Miller, Bruce Larson, Robert Leslie, James Colaianni, and others outside the field of hypnotherapy who have greatly influenced me. Perhaps I will write about their contributions at another time.

I conclude this section with acknowledging the Bible's contributions to Human Trinity Hypnotherapy. The Bible has been the most influential book in my life and it still speaks something new to me each time I read it. The idea of the Human Trinity came from the Bible for there I learned that we are made up of body, mind, and spirit and each affects the others and is effected by the others.

In I Corinthians 3:16, Paul speaks of the importance of the body as he writes, "Know ye not that ye are the temple of God and that the Spirit of God dwelt in you." He speaks of the spirit in I Corinthians 2:9-10, "But as it is written eye hath not seen nor ear heard, neither have entered into the heart of man, the things which God hath prepared from them that love him. But God hath revealed them unto us for his spirit: for the spirit searches all things, yea, the deep things of God." Paul wrote of the mind in II Corinthians 13:11, "Finally, brethren, farewell. Be perfect, be of good comfort, be of one mind, live in peace, and the God of love and peace shall be with you."

Paul continues to write about the human trinity in the twelfth chapter of the book of Romans. Paul writes, "I beseech you therefore brothers by the mercy of God, that ye present your body as a living sacrifice, holy acceptable unto God, which is your reasonable service and be not confined to this world; but be ye transformed by the renewing of your mind, that you may prove what is the good, acceptable, and perfect will of God." (Romans 12:1-2)

In God's sight, the body and the mind as well as the spirit are important. The body is the temple of God, the place were the spirit dwells for Jesus said, "The Kingdom of God is within you." From Paul's verses from Romans, I hear God saying through him that real worship is more than the offering of great prayers. It is more than the offering to God of a ritual, however magnificent. **Real worship is the offering of everyday life to God**.

The renewing of the mind calls for a change in attitude. It calls for us to let go of any negative thoughts because they can be a block to living life to its fullest. God want us to realize our talents, our abilities, our potential, and with divine guidance to use them for our own good and for the good of others. He leads us to look into the heart (subconscious) and mind (conscious) to see our potential and our possibilities rather than our failures and limitations.

In the study of Hypnosis, one can find several references in the Bible to hypnotic like activity. For instance, the first written record of the use of hypnosis is recorded in the book of Genesis 2:21-22, "So the Lord God caused a deep sleep to fall upon man, and while he slept took one of his ribs and closed up its place with flesh, and the rib which God took from man, he made woman and brought her to him." In this incident, God used hypnosis so that Adam felt no pain during the removal of his rib.

Paul speaks of going into a trance while praying in the temple (Acts 22:17). Peter "fell into a trance" and from that experience came to understand that God loves all people and accepts all people who come to him. (Acts 10:1-18) Through the book of Acts, there are a number of references to the apostles looking into the eyes or gazing into the eyes of a person which resulted in the person being healed (Acts 14:9-10). The practice of "laying on of hands" mentioned in the Bible, use some of the techniques of hypnosis (Acts 28:8).

The writer of Proverbs 23:7 said that as a person thinketh in his heart, so is he. St. Paul writes, "Whatsoever a man soweth that shall he also reap." (Gal. 6:7) This says to me that what is sown by the conscious mind through thoughts and images into the subconscious mind tends to become a reality. Mental images gives the subconscious mind a model to work towards. Illustration: Think back to a time when you were very angry. Think back to a time when you were very happy. By thought, you make those feelings present again. The use of positive imagery improves life and health. Until there is an image in the mind, there can by no reality. The author of Proverbs 29:18 also wrote that where there is no vision, the people parish.

In the book of Acts, Chapter 12:2-22, we read the story of Peter being released from prison. King Herod had many of the disciples executed and planned a similar fate for Peter. Peter was arrested and held in maximum security, bound by chains and guarded by two heavily armed guards. Fearing for Peter's life, many people were praying for his well-being and release from prison.

An angel of the Lord appeared to Peter in his prison cell. The angel gave Peter certain instructions of which Peter complied with one step at a time. Following the instructions of the angel, his chains fell off his arms and legs. He put on his sandals and other garments and followed the angel out of the prison. They came to the large iron prison gate and it opened of its own accord. Peter went to the home of a friend realizing that his experience was not an illusion, but he was indeed freed from prison.

To make any Bible story meaningful, we must be able to adopt it to our life situation. First, be reminded that this story has a spiritual and a psychological meaning. There are many people who we counsel who are in a prison of their own making or one which someone else has fashioned for them. It is a prison of anxiety, guilt, grief and pain. Through proper use of hypnotherapy, we can help them be free of their prison cell to a new and better way of life.

Jesus said, "The spirit of the Lord is upon me, because He hath anointed me to heal the broken hearted, to preach deliverance to the captives, and recovery of sight to the blind, and set at liberty them that are bruised." (St. Luke 4:18) Following that guidance and the proper use of hypnosis, we can heal the broken hearted, bring deliverance to those in captivity to pain, fear, and phobias, give sight to the emotionally and spiritually blind, and set at liberty those who are bound by unwanted habits.

(1) Mr. Smith's Case History

I was on my surgery schedule rounds, when I went to visit Mr. Smith. He was scheduled to have his left leg amputated just below the knee. As we visited, Mr. Smith told me that he had been going through many emotional states since learning of the need for surgery. "I felt angry, sad, mad, and disappointed," he said. He went on to talk about his faith and how he had always relied on that in the past, but was having difficulty experiencing the presence of God now.

I told him that the feelings that he was experiencing were natural. I reminded him of Job in the Old Testament and how he questioned his suffering. Job also had difficulty recognizing that God cared for him in his sickness and loses. Job blessed our questions. We can learn something from Job. He questioned but remained opened to God's presence and indeed God came to assure Job of his love and presence.

(2) Man with One Leg

I told Mr. Smith of a devotion which I had read in Guidepost a few days before. In a little town in the French Pyrenees, there is a shrine which is known for its miracles of healing. As the story goes, an amputee veteran of World War II appeared one day at the shrine. As he hobbled up to the shrine, a bystander remarked, "Poor man, does he think God will give him back his leg?" The Veteran overheard him and replied, "No sir,

I don't expect God to give me back my leg. I am going to pray to Him to help me live without it."

Mr. Smith asked me to pray with him for courage to adapt to his amputation and to help him live without his leg. I prayed, "O God I pray with Mr. Smith today as he prepares for surgery and may he know you are with him. I pray for him to be able to make any adjustments he needs to make to live life the best he can with one leg. I pray for his comfort and peace of mind." (As he was an Episcopalian, I continued with this prayer from the Book of Common Prayer), "Almighty God, who did send Thy son, Jesus Christ, to be the Great Physician of our souls and bodies, grant us Thy peace. Thou who givest rest to those who wait upon thee, grant us Thy courage. In quietness and confidence may we find strength. Give wisdom and skill to those who operate and to those who serve as nurses. We give ourselves to Thy sustaining presence, knowing that in Thee is our peace; through Jesus Christ our Lord, Amen."

After we talked for a while, I asked if I might read some Scriptures to him and he said, "yes." I read, "Who shall separate us from the love of Christ? Shall tribulation, or distress, or persecution, or famine, or nakedness or peril or sword? . . . Nay, in all these things we are more than conquerors through him and loved us. For I am persuade that neither life, nor death, nor angels, nor principalities, nor power, nor things present, nor things to come, nor heights, nor depths, or any other creature shall be able to separate us form the love of God in Christ Jesus" (Romans 8:35-39). As I departed, I said, "May God give you peace and comfort for tonight, be with you through the night, be with you through surgery, and bring the strength to make the adjustment you must make. God bless you."

(3) Verses of Help from the Bible

Proverbs

"A wise man will hear and will increase learning; and a man of understanding shall attain wise counsel" (1:5). Happy is the man that findeth wisdom, and the man that getteth understanding. For the merchandise of it is better than the merchandise of silver, and the gain thereof than fine gold" (4:7). Hate stirreth up strifes; but love covers all sins" (10:12). A soft answer turneth away wrath; but grievous words stir up anger" (15:1). "A cheerful heart does good like a medicine, but a broken spirit makes one sick" (17:22).

Psalms

"Give ear to my word, O Lord, consider my meditation. Hearken unto the voice of my cry, my King, and my God; for unto thee will I pray" (5:1-2). "Wait on the Lord; be of good courage, and He shall strengthen thine heart; wait I say, on the Lord" (27:14). "Hear, O Lord, and have mercy upon me; Lord be thou my helper. Thou hast turned my mourning into dancing; Thou has put off my sackcloth and girded me with gladness" (30:10-11). "God is our refuge and strength, a very present help in time of trouble" (46:1). "Cast thy burden on the Lord, and he shall sustain thee" (5:22).

Old Testament

"Thou will keep him in perfect peace, whose mind is stayed in thee; because he trustest in thee. Trust ye in the Lord forever" (Isaiah 26:3-4). "Blessed is the man who trusteth in the Lord, and whose hope the Lord is" (Jeremiah 11:7). "He hath shewed the O man what is good; and what does the Lord require of thee, but to do justly, and to love mercy, and to walk humbly with thy God" (Micah 6:8).

New Testament

"Peace I leave with you, my peace I give unto you, let not your heart be troubled, neither let it be afraid" (John 14:2). "And Jesus looking upon them saith; with men it is impossible, but not with God; for with God all things are possible" (Mark 10:27). "Cast all your cares up on Him (God) for He careth for you" (1 Peter 5:7). "Finally brethren, whatever is true, whatever is honorable, whatever is lovely, whatever is of good report, if there is any excellence and if anything is worthy of praise, let your mind dwell on these things" (Philippians 4:8).

Section Two
Review and Update of Human Trinity Hypnotherapy

CHAPTER SIX

RELEASING ANXIETY AND FEAR

In addition to the Holy Trinity and the Human Trinity, there is an Unholy Trinity. I first heard of the unholy Trinity during an audio seminar by Dr. Daniel Zalling of the Ohio Institute of Medical Hypnosis. Dr. Zalling speaks of the Unholy Trinity as being anxiety, fear, and guilt. I would like to take the liberty of combining anxiety and fear and adding anger. Therefore, the Unholy Trinity consist of (1) anxiety and fear, (2) anger, and (3) guilt.

Throughout history, certain periods or "Ages" have been designated to identify that period. We have had the Stone Age, Ice Age, Bronze Age, Iron Age, the Age of Reason, the Atomic Age, and it could be said that the current age is the Age of Anxiety. We are anxious and fearful about many things. Montarique said, "It is fear that I stand most in fear of." President Franklin D. Roosevelt said to a fear paralyzed nation at the beginning of World War II, "We have nothing to fear, but fear itself."

The days in which we live are interesting, exciting, sometimes thrilling, sometimes disappointing, and sometimes a bit frightening. Everyday we see our scientific knowledge and skills move forward with giant steps. We have spoken proudly and somewhat boastfully of all we have been able to do and accomplish. But if you look carefully, you may notice that many are beginning to tremble like someone holding a time bomb in his hand who doesn't know when it is set to go off. Anxiety and fear seems to be destroying the paradise we have developed here on earth.

One of the problems hampering the building of the Golden Gate Bridge was distinctly human. It was estimated that some 35 lives would probably be lost during the construction. The workmen were filled with increasing fear. Many of them began to worry whether or not he would be among the predicted casualties. Every practical precaution was introduced, but nothing seemed to relieve the anxiety of the workman. It was obvious that their work was affected by the dreadful thought, "What if I should fall into the deadly water below?"

Finally, the chief engineer came to the conclusion that it was the fear of falling rather that the actual probability of falling that troubled the men. If every man had the guarantee that should he fall from the bridge, he would not fall into the deadly water, but would be safely caught, the anxiety would be relieved and his work would improve. The answer was a great net which was hung under the bridge. It cost $80,000 but the expense proved to be a good investment because when the net was in place, the fear of falling was greatly reduced. The men worked faster and more efficiently since they now had a satisfying answer to the troublesome question, "What if I should fall from the bridge?"

The fact of fear is a fact of life. We have fears of the past, present, and future. What if I should lose my job? What if I should lose my health? What if my spouse should leave me? What if I am robbed? What if I should die? These and other questions only add to our anxiety and fear.

Anxiety and fear are destructive agents which prevent us from fully enjoying life. The ancient Vikings had a proverb which might shed some light on this problem. "Vain is the strong oak in our ships without strong hearts in our people." One could paraphrase that proverb with "Vain is the strong oak in our ships when there is fear in the heart of our people." Like a long finger stretching over the centuries, the truth of the proverb is pointing right at one of our weakest points. Vain is all the progress we have made in the material world, the machines we have built, and the power we have harnessed, if we are not able to properly control and use our power. What good are inventions and discoveries, skills and techniques, great learning and extensive education, if one's life is lived in fear.

(1) Strawberry Scarecrow

In an essay, Frank Boreham tells us that as he walked in the country, he came upon a field of strawberries. In the center of the field was a strikingly ugly scarecrow. His arms were stretched out as if to catch any luckless individual or creature who would dare to trespass upon the field that he had been charged to guard. What filled Frank with wonder was this: One bird was sitting on an arm and another on the head of the awful looking scarecrow. They had eaten their fill and would enjoy some more strawberries as soon as their hunger demanded it.

In the same essay, Frank writes of other birds not in the field: Some were perched on the fence and others were in the trees that surrounded the field of strawberries. All of these birds seem to desire the strawberries, but they had not eaten a single berry. Why? Because they were afraid of the terrible scarecrow that stood guard. Our first reaction is to feel that they were very foolish birds, but how often have we been defeated or denied joy in our life because of a scarecrow? Some fears are real, some are scarecrows. It is not so much the reality of life which defeats us as how we perceive reality.

Some years ago, a certain man tried to travel as economically as possible as he crossed the Atlantic by ship. To save on the cost of meals, he took along a large supply of crackers and cheese. When the trip was almost over, a fellow passenger casually asked him why he had not eaten in the dining room? Somewhat embarrassed, the man admitted that in order to save money, he had been preparing his own simple meals in his cabin. Imagine how discouraged he was to be told that the cost of the trip included the meals.

We feel sorry for that man, but there is something else that is more discouraging and sad. It is to make the journey of life, eating one's cracker and cheese in loneliness, sadness, and sorrow, when one could have been feasting at the table of God's rich grace; enjoying all the spiritual blessings that God provides for all his children. Isn't it sad to realize that people go through life living with fear and anxiety. They choose to nibble on the crackers and cheese of an inadequate interpretation of life. Though they are straining, striving, seeking, they are not at peace. Fear and anxiety holds them in captivity.

To be human is to sometimes be afraid. General Patton, a great soldier of World War II, once said, "If bravery is a quality which knows no fear, I have never seen a brave man." Some fears are friends, while others are foes. Some fears are useful, some are abnormal. Some fears are an aid to fulfillment, while others are destructive to our well-being. Normal fear directs us to look both ways before crossing the street. Abnormal fear prevents us from crossing the street or to deny our fears and cross without looking both ways.

Jesus told the story of a ruler who called three servants to come before him and gave each of them a certain amount of money. The first two used their money on profitable ventures and increased the amount. The third man hid the money so its value decreased with the rising cost of living. The ruler returned and asked the servants to give an account of how they used their money. To those who gained money, the ruler said, "Well done, you have been faithful, enter into the joy of the Lord." To the man who had hid his money, the Master said that he must give up that which he had been given. It seems to me that the central teaching point of this parable is neither upon increase or lack of increase, nor reward and punishment, but the central point is on fear and lack of trust.

If the third man in trust had used the money for worthwhile causes and returned empty handed, I believe the ruler would have sent into the joy of the Lord with the other two. His mistake was not having failed to produce, but that his fears were so great that he didn't even begin which is a failure to trust. Because of this man's fear, he was like those birds who sat looking at his strawberries but who had not eaten a single strawberry. He allowed himself to be defeated by a few scarecrows.

The first scarecrow we can identify in this parable is that of the man's own seeming littleness. He did not feel he had the ability or talents to increase what he had been given. It appears that we all began life from this position for the feeling of inferiority is apparently universal.

In those early years, it seems that just about everybody is bigger and smarter. With this perspective, the child spends a great deal of time asking himself, "How can I act so that these giants will like me?" This is the need to be loved, appreciated, complimented, accepted, and recognized. It is natural for us to have these desires but for some people, this need determines how they feel about themselves and the world. This scarecrow of this position is a fear to trust oneself.

Eleanor Sommer tells us that nightmares were part of her life when she was a little girl. When she woke up in the middle of the night trembling and fearful, her mother would come into her room and comfort her. "You are the captain of your own ship. Steer it wherever you choose. Steer it away from bad dreams and toward something beautiful and happy." She said that she was not always successful in changing bad thoughts, but was most of the time, enough of the time to keep following her mother's advice. Her mother's advice was helpful for her throughout her life for she had learned to steer her own ship and trust herself.

A second scarecrow may have been unfavorable circumstance. This life style is typical of a person who in his or her childhood did not experience a proper amount of caring love. Such a child comes to feel that his needs may not be met, so why be considerate of others. As they grow to adulthood, they have difficulty forming meaningful and lasting relationships. The individual has the attitude, "If I had an understanding Lord, if I were in good health, if I lived in a different town, if I were in good health, if I lived in a different job, if I had more talents, if luck was on my side, if I was only appreciated, I could develop myself better. However since these things are as they are, I can not be the person I would like to be." The scarecrow of this position is the fear of others and of circumstances.

The third scarecrow was a mistrust of his Lord. The person who holds this attitude perhaps suffered physical abuse as a child. He may come to feel that his environment not only rejects him, but is hostile to him. He builds a protective shell around himself from which he strikes out at others.

The one who hid his money said to the ruler, "I know you are a hard man, taking what you did not lay down, therefore, I put one over on you and hid the money, here, I returned what you gave me." The scarecrow of this position is a fear of God. The man who did not increase failed because he feared himself, others, and God.

When a person can release fears and experience trust, he can live a more meaningful life. This is a mature stance which permits growth, understanding and meaning. The person sees himself as worthwhile and has respect and concern for others. He recognizes his scarecrows for what they are and enjoys the strawberries.

Some of the fears commonly expressed by clients are fear of flying, heights, falling, needles, failing, rejection, pain, exposure, poor performance in sports, public speaking, responsibility, sexual performance, homosexuality, the unknown, death, contamination, blood, animals, impending danger, water, the dark, open spaces, closed space and loss of control.

A fear becomes a phobia when it reaches the point of being triggered by irrational and unknown factors and when it is experienced often enough to disturb a person's everyday life. People with phobias react uncontrollably and unreasonably to the situation they are afraid of because they do not understand the repressed conflict that causes the intense reaction. It is what the fear represents as an unknown danger, and not just the fear itself, that creates the phobic reaction to it.

With a fear, the client can usually tell when it began. A person has a fear of dogs because he remembers being bitten by a dog when he was 6 years old. A person with a phobia just knows that they are extremely afraid of a dog. Thinking of a dog, seeing a picture of a dog, seeing a dog several blocks down the street can trigger the panic reaction.

There are three main ways to deal with fears and/or phobias: A. Symptomatic Approach, B. Circle Therapy, and C. Desensitization.

A. *The Symptomatic Approach.*

This approach works well with high direct suggestible clients. In effect, the therapist literally suggests the problem away. Example: "You are releasing your fear of dogs as you are becoming more and more comfortable when you see a dog."

By using this approach, no harm can come and it works with a small percentage of people. If the symptom recurs, it may indicate that the fear may need to be approached in a different way.

B. *Circle Therapy.*

Circle Therapy is a very successful therapy dealing with fear. It should not be used with phobias. In the hypnotic state, the client is led to feel the fear. As the fear builds and I notice an abreaction (a venting out which is reflected in facial expressions or body movement), I tell the client to "Feel it, feel it: now take a deep breath, blow out the fear and pass it, let it go, and you go ever deeper into the hypnosis state." I then give positive statements that the next time they feel more comfortable and in control. Again have them experience the fear, let go, feel better. Each time you make the circle, the fear and abreaction is reduced. When it is apparent that the client is letting it go, I say, "Feel it but the harder you try to feel it, the more difficult it becomes to feel it. In fact, you begin to identify an amusement about the situation. You begin to smile and feel at ease." If regression is used or not to find cause, a suggestion such as "Let go of the past, the past cannot affect you now, and the next time this situation occurs, you feel comfortable and relaxed."

Dr. John Kappas states that during Circle therapy, the client faces his fear in a controlled situation of the hypnotic states, which:

1. Weakens the symptoms and allows the client to face it again once the abreaction has ceased
2. Allows the subject to face the cause without experiencing the symptom
3. Increases the subject ability to adopt
4. Can relieve the fear of loss of control and the dread that fear will someday control the subject completely
5. Helps remove the fear of facing the trauma alone
6. Allows for a positive behavior to be substituted for a negative one

C. *Systematic Desensitization.*

Desensitization is very similar to Circle therapy and can be used for either fears or phobias. The main difference between circle therapy and desensitization is that the client is not allowed to fully experience the situation. Using the finger rising technique, have the finger rise as soon as the fear begins to be experienced and let it go, feel calm and relaxed and the repeat. Visualize that you feel calm and relaxed when in a situation that normally causes fear.

In desensitization, I may have the client view the fear from a distance and suggest a feeling of being calm and relaxed. Next, I have the client come closer to the fear and letting go of anxiety and fear. I make a point to face fear in a normal way, because it may be a normal fear that has been exaggerated. To fear a rattle snake is a normal fear. To be so afraid of rattlesnakes that you can't visit your uncle who lives in the country is abnormal.

(2) Martha's Case History

Martha came to me with a fear of flying. I used a desensitization experience with her. Using a finger rising technique, I had her lift her first finger of her left hand as soon as she experienced any fear with the imagery being used. When her finger lifted, I asked her to take a deep breath and as she exhaled to let the fear go, feeling calm, relaxed and at peace. This would be repeated till the fear was released.

(3) Fear of Flying Desensitization

I had her imagine calling the airline and choosing a flight best suited for her schedule, packing for the trip, checking baggage, waiting for boarding, entering the plane, taking off, flying to her destination, landing, and leaving the plane. At each step along the way, when she felt fear, she lifted her finger and let the fear go: feeling calm, relaxed, and at peace. We repeated this until she was able to face the fear in a normal way.

(4) Self-Esteem

I concluded the session with Martha with a Self-Esteem script:

Go deeper now within yourself, relax . . . as I speak to your subconscious mind, know how truly precious and wonderful you are, how important you are to yourself and others. Affirm now, as you go deeper, your desire to feel good about yourself as you become more responsible, honest and loving in all your relationships. It is truly a wonderful feeling to make decisions to increase your feeling of self-worth that help you be a positive and productive person. You have a deep sense of pride and security. As you go deeper now within yourself, relax. Your subconscious awareness expands . . . because you truly love and care about yourself, you take time to think carefully and truthfully before you make any important decisions. You face problems with joy and meet them head-on, knowing you make good decisions which put you actively in charge of your life and leads you on constructive, loving, meaningful paths. It is truly a wonderful feeling to release anger, guilt, grief, rejection and frustration and choose love and commitment.

You joyfully choose to be all that you can be, to share your love, sincerity and commitment with family and friends. You bask in God's love and acceptance, knowing you are a precious child of God and that God loves you. Knowing that God loves you, it easy for you to love . . . for you know that you are loved, that you are loving that you are loved. How powerful that feels! How wonderful! Gratitude fills your body and spirit as you realize you are in charge of your life! And what a wonderful life it is! (I told her Frank Boreman's strawberry field scarecrow story and then continued.)

. . . You have recognized your scarecrow for what it is and can now enjoy the strawberries of flying. You feel good about yourself in a joyful, unselfish manner. You feel good about yourself and you can now enjoy flying.

Go deeper within yourself now, and relax. Just relax. How good it feels to just let go and drift down deeper and deeper as you listen to the sound of my voice. You are confident of the changes you now feel, want and accept for yourself. How happy you are to be responsible and in control of yourself! You are radiant, energetic, confident, and filled with an incredible sense of personal power and freedom . . . isn't it a wonderful feeling to know that you choose positive attitudes and adventures which enhance your well being.

As you look to your future, it is a bright and exciting future. You realize that you have released your fears and its negativity . . . it is truly past, faded, gone. Close the door on the mistakes, fears, and pain of the past as you look to your wonderful, shinning future. You are a productive, honest, caring loving adult. You treat yourself with love and consideration. You make decisions which enhance and better your life and your relationships. You build bridges of strength and confidence one day at a time. You see the scarecrow, recognize it for what it is and enjoy the strawberries. Feeling good about yourself and enjoy your next flight.

I see Martha from time to time and she told me that she is now able to enjoy flying and refers others to me who have a fear of flying. I am happy for her because her job requires that she flies often.

The Bible is a great psychological book as well as a religious book. Jesus knew that the abnormal experiences of fear and anxiety were destructive to health and happiness. Jesus said, "Will your worries and anxieties add a single moment to your life" (Matthew 6:27)? St. Paul wrote, "For God hath not given us the spirit of fear, but of power, and of love and of a sound mind" (II Timothy 1:7). Release your fears and anxieties so that you may be free to live the more abundant life.

Chapter Seven
Releasing Anger and Resentment

The feeling of anger is an emotion which is familiar to each of us. It is a feeling that each of us experiences from time to time and is often justified. I am not saying that you ought not get angry, or be resentful because these are human emotions and therefore OK. It becomes a problem for us by how we react to the anger and whether we control the anger or the anger controls us. St. Paul had great insight when he wrote to the Ephesians "Be angry and yet do not sin; do not let the sun go down on your anger" (4:24).

Something happened to you and you felt angry about it. Perhaps you have held on to it for years so that it has become resentment. The Simonton's in their book *Getting Well Again,* writes, "Resentment is not the same as anger. Anger is generally a single, relatively short-lived emotion, whereas resentment is a long-term process . . . No matter how justified those feelings may have been when the experience first occurred, continuing to carry them has tremendous physical and emotional cost." The only change to that statement I would make is that resentment is anger that is prolonged and continues well beyond the initial experience.

The resentment may have been brought on by childhood abuse, an illness, a financial setback, a broken marriage, a broken friendship, an accident, and the anger continues to affect you in the present. To continue to react with anger leads to a mind that becomes fatigued by the constant physical, emotional, and spiritual drain of that inner conflict. The human heart, mind, and body cannot carry the heavy weight of prolonged or excessive resentment and anger without making the person ill.

Think of the external changes which take place when you get angry: a reddening of the skin of the face, a widening or tightening of the jaw, clenching of the fist and tremor of the voice. Now a good actor can conceal some, if not all these external manifestation, but one cannot stop the effect of the internal changes.

Internally, when a person becomes angry, the muscles of the stomach and intestinal area squeezes down and can cause the digestive tract to become so spastic that one may experience mild to severe abnormal pains. The heart rate increases markedly during anger, blood thickens, blood pressure rises rapidly, and arteries and vessels squeeze down. The worst that can happen is a heart attack or stroke.

In a newspaper article, Paul Roeburn writes that people with heart disease more than double their risk of a heart attack when they get angry, and the danger lasts for two hours. "Others studies have shown that anger increase the heart rate, boost high blood pressure and encourages the clogging of arteries. But this is the first controlled study to find that anger can be an immediate trigger of a heart attach," said Dr. Murray Mittleman.

"Despite the public's impression that outbursts of anger can trigger heart attacks, there hasn't been any scientific evidence to support this. Most physicians thought it was coincidence," said Mittleman. The study was based on 1,122 men and 501 women who had survived heart attacks. It was found that their risks were about 2.3 times higher during the two hours after they got angry. Mittleman said that people who remain calm during emotional conflicts might be able to reduce their risk of a heart attack.

When the suffering man of the Old Testament, Job lost his property, his family, and his health, he became angry with God for his misfortune. Job expressed his anger to God before his friends. The response was, "You can't question God." Job was not afraid to ask "Why?" Nor was he willing to stop with that question, for he struggles through the questions to a greater faith. Those who cannot comprehend why one suffers beyond anything they could deserve will find Job thinking their thoughts.

If I need to ask you a question, but I cannot trust you to accept my question, then I have built a barrier between you and me. I feel that the same thing is true when I have a question for God, but cannot trust him to accept my question. If I cannot trust God to accept my question, how can I trust God to accept me? It is as we are able to trust God to accept us with our questions that we can get beyond the questions to a greater faith.

Let go of your anger and resentment so that your anger no longer controls you. As long as you are angry with a person that person has power over you. To be released from anger and resentment, you need to learn to forgive and release resentment.

A good technique for releasing anger and resentment is to imagine the person you feel angry toward in a chair sitting in front of you. Say to that person, "I forgive you for ________." Following the forgiving exercise, imagine good things happening to that person. Say to that person, "May life's richest blessing be yours." You may find this difficult to do, but keep doing it until you have released the resentment. The purpose of this exercise is to relieve the individuals of the burden of their anger.

(1) Robert's Case History

Following ulcer surgery, a 32-year-old school teacher who I will call "Robert" was referred to me by his doctor for stress management. He reported his problems were tension, nervousness, anxiety, boredom, and lack of energy. During our first session, I asked Robert for his definition of stress. He answered with a description of how he felt. I told him that was common to describe how stress makes us feel instead of a definition. Perhaps the best answer I have ever received was from a woman who responded, "Stress is anything that throws the normal out of balance."

I told Robert that the effect of stress depends on how we react to it rather than the event or experience. I went over several stress management techniques which will be in the chapter on stress management. We concluded the session with a hypnotic induction, progressive relaxation and used a stress reduction and healing script with him.

(2) Calm and Relaxed for Stress Management

As you lie there deeply relaxed, you can let the words "calm and relaxed" repeat themselves in your mind, slowly, softly, soothingly, over and over . . . calm and relaxed . . . now let the words "calm and relaxed" flow down, out of your mind and throughout your entire body, as if they are flowing in your bloodstream, to all parts of your body . . . and wherever those words flow, feeling a strengthening taking pace, as if those words are being absorbed by every cell in your body . . . strengthening, nourishing, calming, soothing . . . feeling stronger and more confident with every passing moment, with every breath that you inhale . . . allow the words "calm and relaxed" to flow throughout your body, feeling and strengthening your body and your mind . . . realizing within yourself that you are now using your own resources to strengthen yourself, enabling you to remain strong and calm even when under stress. All that I'm doing is helping you learn how to focus your concentration for your own benefit . . . and now that you are aware of your ability to strengthen and nourish yourself, this process can continue even when you are not aware of it, just as an underground river continues to flow, strong and sure, even when you are standing on the ground and are unaware of it; just as a flower continues to grow even though you can't see the growth from moment to moment . . . and the growth and strengthening within you continues to develop . . . increasing your self-confidence, self-appreciation, and self-worth. Now allow yourself to experience the freedom to make healthy changes in your life style and accept the opportunity for the future to be different from the past as you progressively improve in all areas of your life.

(3) WARM LIGHT OF HEALING

Imagine, now, that hovering over your body is a globe of bright light; a sphere of warm energy that sends out rays of warmth and healing that penetrates every fiber of your being. You can feel the warmth spreading throughout the totality of your body/spirit/mind . . . this sphere of light and warmth and healing has been sent to you from God who created and maintains the universe . . . these rays are warming you, healing you, penetrating and joining with all that is you . . . now imagine that these deeply warmly relaxing rays are tapping the powers of the universe and are healing and soothing your spirit, mind, and body. Imagine also, that the sphere itself slowly descends upon and into your being, merging with and becoming part of every aspect of your being, such that now the rays radiate outward from you, forming a glowing shield, encircling your essence. It is warming, relaxing, and healing at the deepest level of your being. [Suggestions for relaxation, calmness, and quietness were continually repeated. Post-hypnotic suggestions for calmness, and quietness were continually repeated.]

During the third session, Robert told me that he was having difficulty in maintaining an erection. He would have an erection until he tried to enter, then his penis would wilt. During therapy that day, we did the finger response technique.

(4) FINGER RESPONSE FOR THERAPY

You are relaxed and at ease now, and you continue to feel calm, relaxed and peaceful as I talk to you. You are experiencing the wonderful sensations that relaxation brings to you. You are relaxed and comfortable. In fact, you're becoming more relaxed with each breath you take. With each sound that you hear, you become more and more relaxed. You become more relaxed as you are experiencing a wonderful peace of mind.

There are some questions which I would like to ask you. Now, these questions can be answered "yes" or "no," and I will go no further unless I feel it is important to discuss an area with you to remove any blocks to your subconscious. This will be done only with your consent.

I am going to ask you some questions which can be answered either "yes" or "no." Your subconscious mind is able to answer each question I ask you. You may take a mental journey and let your subconscious respond to the questions.

Your subconscious mind is controlling the fingers of your hand. I request that your subconscious mind pick out a "yes" finger, and that finger is becoming very light. In fact, it is lighter than air and just wants to float up. Don't resist it, don't assist it, just let it drift up. The "yes" finger is beginning to rise. That's good, your first finger of your right hand is the "yes" finger. Now just let your finger float back down, and as it does, you become twice as relaxed.

Now, allow your subconscious mind to pick out a "no" finger. Now, just let the "no" finger began to rise. Your subconscious mind is causing your "no" finger to rise. That's good. Your first finger of your left hand is the "no" finger. Now, just let your finger float back down, and as it does, you become twice as relaxed.

Your subconscious mind is controlling your "yes" finger and your "no" finger. Let us begin with the questions and just let your subconscious answer "yes" or "no."

1. Is there some emotional reason for your problem? *yes*
2. Have you gone through some experience in the past that is causing? *yes*
3. Are you identifying with someone else, perhaps a parent or other significant other who? *no*
4. Are you using the problem to punish yourself? *no*
5. Is this problem related to guilt feeling? *yes*
6. Are you using the problem to punish someone else? *yes*
7. Is there any conflict concerning sex that contributes to your problem? *no*
8. Is this a relationship problem? *yes*
9. Do you experience this problem when you are angry? *yes*
10. Do you experience this problem when you feel stress and tension? *yes*
11. Is it OK with your subconscious mind to get rid of these problems? *yes*

As you will see later, I missed the most important answer to those questions as I focused on question #5 concerning his answer, *yes* in regards to guilt. The majority of erection problems I have dealt with were the result of guilt feelings over some mistake or supposed mistake in the past. But, as you will see, that is not always true.

I worked with Robert for about five months with significant improvement in his health and handling of stress, but no progress with his impotence. One day, Robert came in very mad. Robert said that no matter what he said, his son would take the opposite view. Robert reported that he was most upset because his wife took his son's side in the argument. "It is always like that," he said.

While he talked, I realized that I had missed two important responses to the finger responses to the finger response questions. He had responded *Yes* to the question, "Are you punishing someone else?" *No* to the question, "Are you using this to punish yourself?" and *Yes* to the question, "Is this a relationship problem?" I had failed to recognize that the problem was connected with his feeling toward his wife because he had always idealized that relationship during our sessions.

During the hypnotic session, he said that he was angry with his wife for always siding with their son and impotence was his way of punishing her. I had him visualize his wife sitting in the chair across from him and he was to tell her about his feelings. I then asked him if he could forgive her and he told her that he would forgive her and would she forgive him. He forgave and was forgiven. I then had him picture good things happening to his wife. I then told Robert a healing story about breaking through shells.

(5) Breaking Through Shells with Additional Suggestions for Overcoming Impotence

A few years ago, the cover of the April issue of the religious publication *Daily Word* showed a fluffy golden chick that had just stepped out of a broken shell. As this was the Easter edition, several people wrote *Daily Word* saying that they did not think the cover was religious enough for the occasion. Yet, I wonder if there is anything more religious than a broken shell and a new life rising out of it.

Is there a shell you need to break through today? (You may mention the shell by name.) Sometimes these shells are caused by physical limitation, sometimes emotional limitations, sometimes spiritual limitations and sometimes a combination of any or all three.

The fertilized egg begins to develop a baby chick. By an inner action, growth, and development, the chick begins to grow. It begins to pick at it shell until it breaks and the chick is free. We have within our mind the ability to grow and develop beyond what we had thought possible. By your mental unfolding, you can leave your hurts, disappointments and failures behind and break through your shell.

Think again of the chick breaking out of its shell: a soft, helpless chick begins to pick at the fixed and rigid limits of its world and keeps picking until the limits give way and it is able to stand erect and free. If a little chick can break through such a shell, you can break through your shell. Tonight or tomorrow night, when you began to touch and fondle your wife and are being touched and fondled by her, you respond appropriately and enjoy your time with her. Visualize your penis erect, visualize yourself and your wife enjoying foreplay. As you penetrate your penis remains hard and stiff. You go through the sex act in a loving manner which brings satisfaction to both you and your wife. It is a good experience and you break through your shell.

Robert was scheduled for a session in one week. About two days later, I saw Robert at a local shopping center. When he saw me a big smile came over his face. He said, "First time in two years." I did not have to ask him what he meant.

After the next session, we terminated counseling. He was handling stress appropriately and now understood that by punishing his wife, he was punishing himself. By forgiving his wife and being forgiven, he was now free to enjoy sex. About six months later, he returned with the impotence problem and same cause. He still reverts to old patterns when he subconsciously needs to punish her. Using the same and similar techniques, he is able to overcome his anger and is moving on to a more joyful life. I concluded the last session with a healing script.

(6) Restoring Health

The suggestion and instructions that I'm telling you now are going into the storehouse of your mind and your own mind can cause them to began working immediately in your body . . .

Even though you are not consciously aware of it, the healing processes of your body continues functioning at all times . . . They are continuously nourishing tissues, strengthening muscles, repairing cells, keeping your body temperature stabilized, keeping your heart pumping and causing your blood to continue circulating, cleansing waste material and impurities out of your body through the normal, natural processes of your elimination system, and conducting many other activities . . .

Those processes are continuously working to keep your body healthy and strong . . . They are normal and natural . . . They keep functioning twenty-four hours a day, causing all organs, all glands, all cells, all atoms and molecules of your body to work properly . . .

Scientists have found that each cell of your body performs functions that the world's most outstanding chemists, scientists, and physicians have not been able to duplicate . . . And those activities in your body are guided and directed by your subconscious mind . . . Imprints, impressions, thoughts and ideas have been going into your mind ever since you came into existence, and your mind operates form the accumulation of all the information that is stored there, whether the information is correct or is incorrect.

If the information is incorrect, your mind can review it and understand it now from a more knowledgeable, more mature point of view, and can restore your body to perfect health. This means that your own mind can cause your body processes to function properly and produce healing energies that heal your body perfectly, and you can help your mind to produce proper healing energies by thinking pleasant . . . uplifting thoughts about yourself, and by imagining yourself as being healthy and strong. That causes your mind to activate the processes of your body to renew and rejuvenate every atom, every cell, every organ to include your sexual organs so that they function properly.

The fact that your mind controls your body is not something new. Thomas Edison did research on that subject many years ago, and he discovered that "Every cell of the body thinks." He learned that every cell of the body has a mind and receives directions from the subconscious mind . . . And the Bible says the same thing: It says, "As we think in our heart, so are we." In other words, thoughts and ideas, impressions and imprints made in our mind cause our body to respond, and they can cause us to be sick or healthy, depending on the way our mind has received the information . . . That's the reason our mind can generate the healing chemistry needed in your body, to restore, heal, rebuild, and strengthen your body.

Your subconscious mind has the power to direct the cells to send healing energy through your body and restore your body to health.

The strongest force of energy your body possesses is your own mind . . . and when you have been experiencing illness or disease or any kind of physical handicap, it is possible for change either in body, mind or spirit. Your body may be transformed into a healthy body by renewing your mind with thoughts and ideas of health, confidence, happiness and love . . . That's one of the meanings of the verse in the Bible that says, "You can be transformed by the renewing of your mind." That is what you are doing now. Letting your mind work for you so that you have healthy thoughts and a healthy body . . .

Chapter Eight
Forgiveness and Forgiving

Guilt is a great destroyer of our health and well being: physical, emotionally, and spiritually. Nothing is more meaningful for the human race than our free will, but perhaps nothing is a greater cause of suffering. When one misuses his/her freedom, he/she feels guilty. Guilt cause suffering because it separates us from God, others, and ourselves. It limits our creativity, diminishes our self-worth, creates self-hatred, and casts a shadow over our lives.

After he murdered the king, Macbeth is frightened. Ghosts lurk in dark hallways ready to attack him. He hears a voice crying, "Macbeth will sleep no more." Then a knocking and he cries out in terror, "Whence is that knocking? How is it with me every noise appalls? What hands are here? They pluck out mine eyes." He continues, "Will all great Neptune's ocean wash this blood clean? No, this my hand will rather multitudinous seas incarnadine making the green one red."

Lady Macbeth tells her husband to throw off his fears. She appears to be so strong in the face of their evil deed! Her strength leaves her and in the last act her nerves give away. She walks at night in a daze. Her nurse watches her wash her hands again and again as she cries, "Out damned spot!" More washing and "Here's the smell of blood still: All the perfumes of Arabia will not sweeten this little hand." Watching from a corner, the physician says, "Foul whisperings are abroad; unnatural deeds do breed unnatural troubles; infected minds to there deaf pillow will discharge their secrets; more she needs the divine than the physician. God, God forgive us all!"

Though guilt is a destroyer of our well-being, it has positive as well as negative qualities. The positive aspect of guilt is that it is to spiritual and emotional health what pain is to physical health. It is a warning that something is wrong and that a change of some kind is necessary for wholeness.

Like physical pain, the intensity of guilt is not necessarily an indication of how serious the wrong may be. For instance, a hangnail may be more painful than certain stages of cancer. The same is true of guilt. Many of us carry throughout our life an unnecessary weight of guilt for relatively small mistakes or even supposed mistakes. On the other hand, the absence of the discomforting feeling of guilt may not be a necessary sign of spiritual and emotional health.

So often unresolved guilt (whether real or imaginary) creates a need to make amends, to make restitution, to suffer enough to pay back the wrong, to set things right by damage, to self and thus to balance the account. An accident-prone person may be punishing himself for real or imagined sins. By having a car wreck, cutting his hand, or falling down, the person may be punishing himself. A failure-prone person maybe a failure because she/he believes subconsciously that she/he is not worthy of success.

Our guilt which results in a failure to find peace within ourselves is the cause of many of our physical illnesses and injuries. There are many illnesses that come as the results of germs and physical malfunction which are no fault of our own, but there are also a number of illnesses and injuries which results from guilt.

Many physicians are on record as stating that over 50% of our illnesses have their origin in our minds and spirits. In other words: germs, physical malfunction, and unpreventable accidents do not cause half the trouble that comes from guilt, nervous tension, emotional stress, and spiritual unrest. Our disturbing sense of guilt and deep rooted fears play havoc with our health and well-being.

Habitual grudges, resentment, smoldering rage, the war within weakens our body's resistance to disease and/or leads one to carelessness which results in an accident. A recent newspaper article by a medical doctor stated more heart trouble is caused by inner tension, guilt, and resentment than are caused by smoking, drinking, or fatty substances in the blood.

There is an interesting passage in *Gone With The Wind* at the funeral of General O'Hara. His prospective son-in-law said something like this, "There wasn't nothing that came to him from the outside that could lick him . . . but he had his failings too, cause he could be licked from the inside."

Bernard de Clairivaux said centuries ago, "Nothing can cause me damage except myself." Remember the words of Cassus to Brutus in *Julius Caesar,* "The fault, dear Brutes, is not in our stars but in ourselves." These statements and other evidence leads me to believe that there are only two ways to deal with guilt. Guilt, whether real or imaginary, must either be forgiven or punished. It is not God who punishes us, but we find a way to punish ourselves. We need to experience God's forgiveness and forgive ourselves.

(1) Lou Gehrig Strikes Out

In New York City, a sports writer was deeply impressed by an incident involving the baseball player Lou Gehrig. In typical sports jargon he wrote that Lou Gehrig came to bat with two out in the ninth inning. The run to tie the game was on third and the winning run was on second. New York was one run behind and a hit would either tie the score or win the game. The count on Lou Gehrig went to three balls and two strikes. The people in the stands were in an uproar. The pitcher wound up deliberately and the third strike came smoking in straight over the middle of the plate and the umpire shouted, "Strike three!" Lou Gehrig had not moved his bat. Very slowly Lou turned, spoke to the umpire and walked to the bench. At that, the crowd went wild for no one had ever seen Lou Gehrig argue with an umpire. The reporters all piled over the seats and right out onto the field. They swarmed around the umpire. The writer asked, "What did Lou Gehrig say to you? Whatever it was will make the headlines on the sports page." The umpire smiled and yelled to Lou Gehrig to come over. He said to Lou, "Tell the boys what you said to me when I called the third strike on you." Lou looked a little bewildered as he answered, "Mister Ump, I only said, 'I would give ten dollars to have that one back'."

The reporter was so impressed that when he wrote the story, he added, "There are people all over the world who would give ten dollars or ten thousand dollars to get just one minute back and for the privilege of changing something they said or did in that minute."

One cannot change a past mistake, a lost opportunity, a hurting word, but one can experience forgiveness. Yes, forgiveness, if not from the one harmed, at lease from God. With that forgiveness we can begin again, we can be renewed, we can live more abundantly.

I often use the "finger response to therapy" in dealing with many problems. Using this therapy, I have the clients subconscious mind pick out a "yes" finger and a "no" finger. When the subconscious had decided on a "yes" finger and a "no" finger, I ask questions which can be answered "yes" or "no." It is surprising the high percentage of people who raise the "yes" finger to the question, "Are you trying to punish yourself by this behavior" (smoking, overweight, phobia reaction, etc.) and to the question, "Is this problem the result of guilt feelings?" The individual needs to forgive himself and accept the forgiveness which God has already given.

Most of us are familiar with the story of the Prodigal Son (Luke 15:11-25). The prodigal son expected to be rejected by his father. He prepared a speech requesting that he be accepted as a servant. When the son returned, he was accepted. He was not even able to finish his prepared speech of repentance for the father had already forgiven him. The son was forgiven, but until he returned home, he could not be aware of, or accept, or be made whole by forgiveness. You too can leave the heavy weight of your guilt behind. You are forgiven, now forgive yourself. You have released your guilt though forgiveness; now, you are free to experience a fuller happier life.

In order to experience wholeness, we must not only accept our forgiveness, but we must forgive those who have harmed us. We need to forgive even when the person who has harmed us does not ask for nor deserves our forgiveness. We need to forgive in order to free ourselves of the power the other person has over us. This is especially true of abuse whether it be sexual, emotional, or physical abuse.

The parable of the prodigal son is really the parable of the prodigal sons. The elder son who stayed with the father refused to welcome his younger brother home, refused to forgive him, refused to join the homecoming party. The elder's sons failure to enjoy the brother's party was not the fault of the father. As he welcomed the younger son, the father went out to meet his elder son and invited him to the party. The problem was with the elder son. The older brother was out of fellowship with his brother and his father, he refused to enter the party. He refused to forgive, or to be forgiven and so missed the joy of the occasion.

(2) Sandy's Case History

Sandy is a 21-year-old lady who had been sexually abused by an older brother, who was seven years older than she. She could not be free until she could forgive him. He had not asked her for forgiveness nor was he visibly sorry for his abuse. The forgiving act of this young lady did not change her brother, but it did change her. It took about seven sessions for her to forgive him, but she was finally able to do so.

Though she was very religious, she believed that God was a very judgmental being. This made it difficult for her to experience forgiveness for the false guilt she felt about her sexual experiences with her brother. After this story, she was able to accept God's forgiveness and forgive herself.

(3) Boy Who Refused to Eat Prunes

While she was in a state of hypnosis, I said that as I listened to your description of your upbringing and early religious training, I am reminded of the mother who served stewed prunes for desert one night for her family. When her son refused to eat his prunes, she said, "God does not like that, God doesn't like little boys who don't eat their prunes. God will be very angry."

In spite of his mother's warning, the boy refused to eat the prunes so she sent him to bed saying, "You have been very bad and God is very angry with you." A short time later he went to bed and a terrible thunderstorm broke out: lightening flashed, thunder roared, the wind whipped rain against the window. The mother thought that the boy would be terribly frightened so she went up to comfort him. When she entered the room, he was standing at the window with his face pressed against the glass, saying, "My, my such a fuss over a few prunes." You have often heard that God was angry with you and so it has been difficult for you to feel forgiven and comfortable with yourself and life. God loves you and forgives you, so now it's time for you to accept that forgiveness and forgive yourself.

During that session she forgave herself but it took about three more sessions before she was ready to forgive her brother.

(4) Forgiveness

Sandy, forgiveness is important to your mental, emotional and spiritual well-being. I cannot do this for you, but you can do it. Though I can not do it for you, I can help you allow the forgiveness to be experienced. To help you do this, I would like to lead you through some releasing and forgiving experiences. Is that all right with you? *Yes.* (If not OK, ask, "Why?" If client is not willing to do the exercises, respect their wishes. If OK, continue.)

There is an old Emmet Fox exercise for dissolving resentment that can be helpful. It may be difficult, but let it happen. As you sit quietly with your eyes closed, allow your mind and body to relax even more. Imagine yourself sitting in a darkened theater. In front of you on a small stage, is your brother. When you see your brother clearly, visualize good things happening to him. Things that would be meaningful to him. See him smiling and happy. Hold this image for a few minutes, then let it fade away. Add another step. As he leaves the stage, put yourself up there on the stage. See good things happening to you. See yourself smiling and happy. Be aware that the abundance of the Universe is available for you.

Forgiveness is important but for some of us, there is a step that is necessary before we can totally forgive. Sometimes the little kid in us needs to have revenge before it is free to forgive. Sitting quiet and peacefully, think of your brother (the person who is hardest to forgive). What would you like to do to him? What does he need to do to get forgiveness? Imagine that happening. Get into the details. How long do you want him to suffer or do penance? When you forgive lift your "yes" finger. As you forgive let it go. Be free of the power your brother has held over you. As you forgive, you are free to enjoy life . . .

In your imagination, you are sitting in a chair on the stage in front of your brother. Now prepare to forgive him even if he does no request forgiveness or deserves forgiveness. Say, "I forgive you brother for the sexual things you did to me as we were growing up." She continued on her own, "I forgive you Robert. In so doing, I release myself from the power that you have had over me. That power made me feel guilty, has prevented me from fully enjoying sex with my husband, and has weakened my self-esteem. I am now free to live my life joyfully." I concluded this session with a script on female sexual enhancement.

(5) Female Sexual Enhancement

You are now ready to experience changes in your sexual experience. You choose to leave all past sexual experiences behind you . . . You choose to focus your attention on your new sexual expressions . . . Begin to imagine them now. You are free to be experience sex with your husband and to feel everything you want to feel.

Imagine that you are with your husband . . . You touch him feeling his excitement. You feel his gentle touch raising your sexual feelings . . . You are capable of sexual pleasure and your mind and body enjoys the arousing overtures within you. You enjoy being touched and touching your husband . . . You feel all the pleasure zones of your body and mind growing with excitement. You feel excited when touched and are touching. You are delighted with your sexual arousal. Your breathing increases as you feel more and more exciting sexual stimulation.

Your pleasure is satisfying as it continues to ascent, filling you with enjoyment. Your relationship develops mutual satisfaction. You feel the tender and gentle touch of your husband bringing you to new heights of arousal. Your pleasure mounts higher and higher . . . Your body responds with tingling sensations.

You feel your oneness, your togetherness, your connecting intimacy as your pleasure mounts . . . Your closeness assists your increase of pleasure . . . You feel throbbing stimulation within your body . . . Your pleasure heightens and you burst forth with excitable orgasmic pleasure as your husband responds joyfully. Your climax increases and you feel totally satisfied . . . You feel so good as you have responded naturally and beautifully to your sexual experience which enhances your husband's pleasure also . . . You enjoy your new, more enjoyable, more sexually active life . . . It is good and you deserve it.

Sandy lives a much happier life and responds joyfully during sexual relations with her husband.

In a summary on forgiveness, Dr. Louis Bauer said, "Forgiveness is an act of the will not of feeling, but the good feeling will follow as a by-product. It is in forgiving and being forgiven that we have the key which unlocks the door to wholeness." Dr. Maxwell Maltz concluded his book, *Creative Living For Today* with this statement, "Drink in the sweetness of forgiveness: of yourself and others. You must forgive a parent, a friend, a loved one, for the errors of the past. Forgive the hurt they caused you. Forgive it by loving in the present . . . Now."

Chapter Nine
Releasing the Past

The past pays a tremendous part in what we do, feel, think and how we act. You cannot change the past for it has been lived, but you can change your attitude toward the past so that it can no longer control your present. The past will remain an influence, but you are in control.

When St. Paul wrote, "Forgetting those things which are behind and reaching forth to those things which are before," he was saying that life is for growth, for development, for progress. If you are controlled by the past, life becomes stagnate, bitter, restricted. When I speak of "releasing the past," let us understand that we don't want to get rid of the memory of the past. Many wonderful experiences of the past are part of our memory. Many learning experiences are part of our memory. Using memory correctly helps us meet the needs of today. The past we want to release are those experiences which prevent us from fully living today.

Some people glory in the past as if it was some golden age which will never return. With such an attitude, we live in the fantasies of yesterday and refuse to move up to the realities of today. Others have such an unhappy past that they are continually reacting to life in the here and now on the basis of past hurts.

"I am now what I am because of the past" is the most commonly used reason by which we deny ourselves and others the luxury of growth and change." There is an old saying, "You can't teach an old dog new tricks." The determinist in religion, philosophy, and psychology content that this statement is true, not only of dogs, but also people. The determinist in religion says that our lives are predetermined by God to be what we are. We do not have any say in the matter for we are simple puppets who are played by God's manipulation. The determinist in philosophy and psychology says that our environment, inheritance, and instincts determine us to be what we will be.

Any of these schools of determination leaves a very hopeless and dismal picture to complete. If we are determined to be as we are, then we have no responsibility for a better life. God, heredity, instinct and or environment are the causes of our problems. We can say, "The devil made me do it or God made me do it or my determinism made me do it, I am not responsible."

So your past has left scars. Perhaps you were physically, emotionally or sexually abused as a child and you have been reacting out of that hurt of your life in the present. Perhaps you failed at something in the past and you refuse to move beyond that failure to newness of life. To continue to live in the past is to allow the past to control your actions and attitude today. On the other hand, if we believe that people can release the power of the past and make changes out of their free will then there is HOPE.

When we refuse to move on beyond the past, and worry about yesterday, we waste the strength we need for today. In his autobiography, Milton Berle, once king of night time T.V., shares with the public a portion of his life for the first time. Berle wrote that 40 years before he wrote his book, that he had fathered a child out of wedlock, but had never talked about it before. Berle states, "That was one of the biggest hurts in my life. I got sick over that for years. I had ulcers, sick enough to die, maybe by holding it all in."

We are all confronted with the problem of pollution in our society. If the well documented evidence of pollution in our environment causes you to feel indignation, then consider what is happening in our minds and bodies as a results of polluted thoughts and feelings. Mental pollution is basically filling ones thoughts with the negative. We keep dumping polluted thoughts from the past into our understanding of today. Every time we hold on to anger from the past or hold hateful thoughts or reinforce negative feelings, we are polluting the waters of our mind. Emotional responses of hate, angers, envy, jealously, resentment, guilt, and fear are pollutants that disrupt our lives.

(1) No Dumping Allowed

I share with you an adaptation of a story by Charles Roth: Think of your thoughts as a stream. A life-giving stream . . . that empties out into the field and orchards of life . . . You want to keep that stream pure and fresh . . . Just as nearly pure as when it emerged from its source . . . Because you know you would reap the results of a good harvest in your field and orchards . . .

Your personal world depends on your stream of thought for its prosperity, its health, its beauty, and harmony . . . Just as the farmer's field depends on pure unpolluted water for its maximum yield . . . Begin now today . . . to stand watch over your personal stream of thought. When you find yourself beginning to entertain negative thoughts or emotions be quick to say to yourself, "Sorry, no dumping allowed." (Author's note: Though I normally do not use negative statements in my suggestions, I feel in this case, it is permissible because it is a common sign in our society.)

Some of the techniques that I use to help people release the past are prayer, hypnosis, relaxation, imagery and healing stories. William James once wrote, "The greatest discovery of my generation is that human beings can alter their lives by altering the attitude of their mind." A beautiful woman lay in the hospital with a seriously painful injury. A friend came to visit her. As the friend came to the bedside of the young woman, she had a sorrowful expression on her face. She placed her hand on the young woman's hand and said, "Honey, I'm so sorry for you, for you are in so much pain. I don't know why you have to go through this, for suffering colors your life so much." The young woman smiled at her concerned visitor and replied, "Yes, but I shall choose the color."

What the young woman tells each of us is that we can choose the color, we can choose the bleak colors or we can choose the brighter colors. We cannot always choose what happens to us, but we can choose the attitude we take toward what happens to us.

By the use of our mind, we can use visualization and imagine what we want to happen as if it has already happened and our subconscious mind will begin to work to bring it to reality. One of the great ministers of the century, Dr. Harry Emerson Fasedrick once wrote, "Picture yourself as defeated and that alone will make victory impossible. Picture yourself vividly as winning and that alone will contribute immensely to success. Great living starts with a picture held in your imagination of what you would like to do or be."

(2) Ralph's Case History

Ralph, a 50-year-old male, was unable to let go of an experience from his past. While he was growing up, Ralph went to a Catholic school. He said, "They put the fear of God in me and I resented them for it." Another boy wrote on the bathroom wall, "God is no good." Ralph said that when he read it he felt the same way. As he was walking out of the bathroom, he felt as if he had written the words on the bath room wall himself.

Over the years, he developed a great fear of God. He made a proper living for his family, but could never stay in a job for long. In one session, I told him the story of the little boy who refused to eat prunes. I followed that by telling him that he could look at his experience in the bathroom from another point of view. He could also begin to change his view of God, but, of course, that was his decision to make. He responded that he would like to know a God of love. I said remember the words from St. John (3:16), "For God so loved the world that he gave his only begotten son that whosoever belieth on him should not perish, but have everlasting, life." Release those old negative ideas about God and live in the present with a new understanding.

(3) SHEEP THIEF

Two young men stole some sheep. They were caught and brought to trial. The punishment for the crime was the branding of the initials "S.T." (sheep thief) on their foreheads. One boy left the town and was never heard from but the other remained. As the years passed, he became a man of faith and gave his life to people in love and service.

Many years later, a visitor came to the town and asked an old man, "What does 'S.T.' stand for on the head of that man down the street?" The old man knew the story, but answered, "It happened a long time ago, I have forgotten the details, but for those of use who know him now, it is the abbreviation for the word "Saint."

Yes, change can take place. We do not have to stay the way we are. Some may say, "I wish there were some wonderful place called the *Land of Beginning Again,* where all our mistakes and all of our heartaches and all of our selfish grief could be dropped like a shabby coat at the door and never put on again." Faith says that there is an opportunity to begin again, for through faith you can change as you accept a new vision of what life can be for you. Let the past go. Let old thought patterns be released. Move past the old barriers to a new life.

(4) INVISIBLE BARRIERS (ADOPTED FROM HAVERS AND WALTERS)

(Used for opening life to new experiences and understanding by moving beyond our invisible barriers.) I wonder if you are familiar with fences . . . especially the electric fences used with horses . . . These fences have a few tiny strands of wire and through that wire goes a current of electricity . . . The kind of electricity that is safe; just the kind that gives you a jolt—like static electricity you get from walking on rugs. A sudden, sharp spark . . . these wires stretch all around the field . . . and as the horses walk from place to place . . . they quickly learn where they can go, and where they don't want to venture. All it takes is a few brushes against the wire . . . a few sudden, startling zaps . . . and being very smart animals they learn to look but not to touch . . . They learn so well, in fact, that after a while . . . the farmer can turn off the electricity . . . or even replace the wires with string . . . and those horses will stay put . . . fenced in by nothing at all . . . stopped in their tracks by a thought . . . by the feeling that some places are off limits . . . that where they are is safe . . . as long as they just stay put . . . satisfied to be where they are.

An invisible barrier or boundary can be created by the mind, but once a horse goes through it . . . then he is free to roam as he wishes. You have been bound by the barrier of a 10-year-old boy's thoughts . . . walk through that barrier to freedom from the past . . . You are now an adult and you are beginning to experience God's love for you.

(5) Grandma, Snoopy, and Dancing

My Grandma Sanders was one of the most reflective persons of the love of God that I have ever known, but Grandma had her hangups. I remember spending the night with my grandparents many years ago. During that visit my Grandpa played his french harp. It was a very special evening and it stands out in my memory.

During the evening, my Grandpa played a snappy little tune called, "Soldier's Joy." When he completed the song, my Grandma said, "I don't like that song!" I quickly asked, "Why Grandma? It is a beautiful song." Laughingly, she responded, "I have seen it danced to too often." I don't resent my Grandma for that statement, because she was joking and in a way she was reflecting 65 years of her cultural history. It does bring to mind how much some have missed because they could not dance.

We live in a world where there is hunger, war, crime, sickness, and alienation. Yet in spite of this, we believe that life is worth living and that life is meant to bring love, friendship, understanding, and joy. Contrary to popular belief, the life which God desires for us is not one of denying worthwhile pleasure or of despising basic human satisfaction, but rather one of enjoying our earthly life.

We honor God not by renouncing life, but by joining our spirits with God's Holy Spirit to know and live life at its best. Then, we can give thanks in offering our faith to God, in sharing of fellowship with people in work in play, in laughter and in tears, in health and in sickness, in everything. Through faith, we can dance the dance of joy. David wrote in Psalm 30, "O Lord, Thou has turned my lament into dancing, thou has stripped off my sack cloth and clothed me with joy."

The Snoopy of Peanuts is often leaping and dancing for joy. On one occasion, Snoopy beings to dance about and shouts, "To dance is to live." In the next frame, he says, "I feel sorry for people who cannot dance." In the next frame, he goes on dancing joyfully and says to us, "If you can't dance, at least be able to do a happy hop." I would like to add one more frame, which shows Snoopy continuing to dance and saying, "If you can't dance with your feet, at least be able to dance in your heart." That to me is a picture of wholesome living.

Though Ralph had gone to church all his life, he discovered that for the first time he was enjoying going to church. He accepted God's love for him and began to dance in his heart.

(6) Lot's Wife

Holding on to the past can be destruction to our present well being. In the Old Testament, there is a story about the problems created by holding onto the past (Genesis 19). In the early morning, an angel came to Lot and said, "Arise, take your wife and your two daughters who are here, lest you be consumed in the punishment of the city." Some men lead Lot, his wife, and two daughters out of the city. They told Lot, "Flee for your life; do not look back or stop anywhere in the valley. Flee to the hills, lest your die."

As the group was moving toward the hills, Lot's wife looked back and she became a pillar of salt. The story of Lot's wife is an extreme example of one who refused to let go of the past. Because Lot's wife would not let go of the harmful parts of her past, even under the emergency of the destruction of the cities of Sodom and Gomorrah, she suffered not only mentally but physically. Because she could not let go of the past, she missed her opportunity to start a new life in the present.

(7) Barnacles on the Ship

Our holding on to the past is kind of like barnacles on a ship. Barnacles are a problem for all ocean-going vessels. Those small living creatures attach themselves to the hull of the ship. As they accumulate and grow larger, they not only add to the weight of the boat, they increase the amount of resistance as the boat moves through the water. They add weight to the ship and eventually slows the speed of the boat, decreasing its mobility, and increasing its use of fuel.

As the barnacles grow larger and larger and increases in numbers, the speed of the ship is reduced until, if allowed to remain indefinitely, the barnacles will disable the ship completely. Because of this, the owner of the ship will periodically remove the ship from the water and have the barnacles scraped off the hull.

As we sail through life, we too collect barnacles. We acquire them in our mind. These barnacles are negative attitudes, unfounded fears, feelings of limitations, and incorrect thought patterns. In short, they are anything which mentally weights us down and interferes with our present well being. The more barnacles of the past we acquire, the slower the unfolding of the full life. These barnacles significantly slow us down and impede our progress: physically, mentally, and spiritually. It is up to us to periodically scrape off the barnacles of unwanted beliefs, fears, and negative thinking so we can move forward, unburdened by the extra weight of the past.

We are influenced by our past, but we are not bound by our past. We can change our thoughts about the past in order to experience present growth. We can change the direction of our thoughts and by doing so change our life. Let go of adverse and negative conditioning from the past and refuse their control over your life today. Live life abundantly.

Chapter Ten
A Time to be Active: A Time to be Still

The Bible has many interesting stories, most of which points to a truth beyond the first impression. As a Hypnotherapist and hospital Chaplain, I find the story of Jesus visiting Mary and Martha to be one of those stories that goes beyond appearances. The story found in Luke 10:38-42 has nothing to do with hypnosis . . . or does it? On the surface, this is the record of Jesus visiting Mary and Martha who with their brother, Lazarus, were close friends of Jesus.

While Jesus visits, he begins to talk with the family and other guests. Mary sat at Jesus' feet and listened to every word that he spoke. Martha was busy preparing a meal for Jesus and the others. She comes to Jesus and ask him to tell Mary to help with the preparing of the meal. Jesus responds, "Martha, Martha, you are anxious and worried about many things. Mary has chosen a good part which shall not be taken from her."

You may be wondering, "What does this story have to do with hypnosis?" I would like to approach this story of Mary and Martha from a different stance than its traditional interpretations. Instead of seeing Mary and Martha as two different types of people, let us see Mary and Martha as two parts of our individual personality. There are times that we need to stop, relax, open our minds to new learning opportunities and at other times we need to be active and doing. Perhaps the message of this story is that in order to be our best when doing, we need to just stop, relax, and renew. Is not that what we do during hypnosis?

In the Biblical story of Mary and Martha, Mary had her priorities in order. She had chosen properly. She wanted to hear what Jesus had to say so she sat herself at the Lord's feet to hear him speak. As she was sitting at his feet, eye fixation was established and Mary was open to the good, positive, helpful suggestions of Jesus. She was open to new learning, new understanding, and meaning for new life.

To the Martha in us, Jesus says that there are times when it would have been better for us to just stop and listen. Martha's problem was that she did not have her priorities in order. Jesus is saying that there are times when we need to stop and listen. It is as the Psalmist wrote, "Be still and know that I am God" (Psalm 46:10).

We can learn a lot from Mary for we need to be able to sort out our priorities in life and put first what really counts. Mary teaches us an important lesson about stopping, relaxing, focusing, and listening.

(1) Cindy's Case History

Having been referred to me by her physician, Cindy (a 28-year-old female, married to her third husband with no children) came to me for pain management. As a result of her pain, Cindy stayed in bed most of the time, but would have periods of energy when she was very active. She talked a lot and many of her friends felt that she dominated their conversations. Cindy reminded me a lot of Mary and Martha. She was anxious and troubled about many things, but very responsive to hypnosis.

The first few sessions were used to help her develop self hypnosis and pain management. She was able to reduce her pain considerably and became much more active in her community. Her favorite pain management imagery was that of imagining Jesus by her; visualizing him physically by her and placing his hand on her back. She could feel the warmth, the healing, the easing, of discomfort. She would then allow the physical presence of Jesus in her imagery to fade into a spiritual presence whose touch remained with her after hypnosis. She also was able to use glove anesthesia and transfer the numbness from the hand to the area of pain.

Cindy has very low self esteem and self confidence. After a few sessions, we began to work on these areas. She had to have everything in her house just right. Everything has its place and had to be in place or she would get upset. She was constantly fighting a fear of failure and had a great need to be accepted by others.

(2) Increasing Self-worth: You Are Somebody

Everyone wants to be somebody. Everyone needs to find a personal identity, a meaning for existence, a reason for living. You are learning that you are somebody. Billy Graham tells the story of a farmer's prize pig. The farmer gave the pig a bath, polished his hoofs, put some perfume on the pig and brought it into the house as a pet. Everything was OK until someone left the door open and the pig got outside. Once outside, he jumped into the first mud puddle that he could find. The farmer has cleaned the pig, but he had not changed the fact that he was still a pig.

You are a human being. Unlike the pig who could not change his nature, you can move beyond your old ways of thinking and acting to live a more abundant life. God made you and me. Therefore, love yourself for you are a being of great worth. A worthy self-image has enabled people to conquer prejudice, overcome fatigue, lift depression, break destructive habits, overcome worry, fear, and anxiety, generate enthusiasm, break boredom, overcome the compulsive need to be doing something. So love yourself and feel good about yourself. Your self-confidence and self-worth are increasing, enabling you to make decisions wisely and confidently. Your concentration keeps improving more and more each day, enabling you to set priorities for work and relaxation.

You radiate a very pleasant personality and find your talents, skills, and abilities keep increasing day by day. The subconscious level of your mind causes your creative abilities to keep emerging, enabling you to live to the best of your abilities. You enjoy greater and greater peace of mind as you take time to relax and be at peace. You are somebody and you experience a deep feeling of pride. You are a person of great worth and that feels good.

During age regression, Cindy went back to age five. Her mother was kicking her and screaming at her, "Stupid, stupid." The little girl Cindy kept crying, "I didn't do anything wrong, I am a good girl." I asked her if she needed to go back further in time to the cause of her problem and she nodded, *yes.* "I feel that I am in a black hole. I am afraid. My mother does not want me. She wants me to come out, but I am afraid to. If I come out what will she do with me?" (In a previous session, Cindy had shown me some drawings. All of those drawings had a tornado or black hole in the drawing.) This went on for sometime and concluded with her birth.

Cindy's Initial Sensitizing Event (ISE) was the experience for not being wanted while she was still in her mother's womb. Her Symptom Producing Events (SPE) was the beating by her mother at age five, and the Symptom Intensifying Event (SIE) was a divorce shortly after her first marriage which verified for her that she had no worth. (ISE, SPE, and SIE will be discussed in Chapter 24—Age Regression).

I would like to share with you some of the suggestions, imagery and healing stories used with Cindy, over a three month period. I still see Cindy from time to time at community events and she is much happier, less inhibited by pain, and feels much better about herself as a person.

As Cindy was very responsive to religious imagery, I told her the story of Mary and Martha. I asked her to close her eyes and let the Mary part be still so she could help the Martha part. Cindy just let the Mary part of you take over and just listen. The Psalmist said, "Wait on the Lord, be of good courage and he shall strengthen your heart. Wait, I say on the Lord" (Psalm 27:14). The Psalmist said, "Be still and know that I am God" (Psalm 46:10).

Now listen to the words of Jesus from Matthew 6:25-34.

> *"For this reason I say to you, do not be anxious for your life, as to what you shall eat, or what you shall drink: nor for our body, as to*

what you shall put on. Is not life more than food, and the body than clothing? Look at the birds of the air, that they do not sow, neither do they reap, nor gather into barns, and yet your heavenly Father feeds them. Are you not worth much more than they? And which of you by being anxious can add a single cubit to his life's span? And why are you anxious about clothing? Observe how the lilies for the field grow: they do not toil nor do they spin, yet I say to you that even Solomon in all his glory did not clothe himself like one of these. But if God so arrays the grass of the field, which is alive today and tomorrow is thrown into the furnace, will He not much more do so for you, O men of little faith? Do not be anxious then, saying, what shall we eat? or What shall we drink? or with what shall we clothe ourselves? For all these things the Gentiles eagerly seek: for your heavenly Father know that you need all these things. But seek first His kingdom and His righteousness: and all these things shall be added to you. Therefore do not be anxious for tomorrow; for tomorrow will care for itself. Each day has enough trouble of its own."

From John 14:27 we hear Jesus say,

> *"Peace I leave with you, my peace I give unto you, not as the world gives, give I unto you. Let not your heart be troubled. Neither let it be afraid."* I counted her out of hypnosis and concluded the session.

At another occasion, I told her this story for improving health. This story was written by Audrey "Tucker" Morgan titled, *The Magic Brook.*

(3) The Magic Brook (by Audrey "Tucker" Morgan)

By a lovely tree in the country, there was a gentle brook. It was so cool and fresh and clean. All the animals like to come and drink out of the brook.

Sitting in a blue robe and brown slippers was a wise old man. His hair was silver white and hung to his shoulders. He also had a white beard that fell down into his lap. He had a gentile smile that put everyone at ease. The grownups called him, "The Wise One."

If you drank the water from the brook they would say, "You never get sick." All the grownups brought their children to the brook to drink the water. The Wise Old Man would smile and tell everyone, "Hello."

As the children grew up they noticed that no one got sick. They were all well, not a stomach ache, nothing.

One day a young girl approached the brook alone. The wise old man sat under the tree. He looked at the girl and smiled. The young girl said, "Excuse me, sir, but can you tell me why no one gets sick? If we just drink the water from this brook, we are forever well."

The wise old man smiled and in a very gentle voice said, "The brook has no magic to it." Then he told the girl, "The people believe the brook has the magic to keep them well. Therefore, they don't get sick." The wise old man said, "It's what you believe in your heart that works. There is no magic in the brook, only what's in your heart." Now Cindy, allow the healing powers which God created in you begin to work for your healing and well being; physically, emotionally, and spiritually.

Toward the end of her counseling session, I had Cindy hold the child of her past, love it, and give her the love she did not experience as a baby and little girl. Give the little girl of your past the love she missed as a child. Cindy would cradle the imaginary child of her past, pet it, love it, and tell her how much she loved her.

I concluded Cindy's last session with this story, *Tadpoles and Frogs.*

(4) Tadpoles and Frogs

The Psalmist once wrote, "When I consider thy heavens, the works of thy fingers, the moon and the stars, which thou hast ordained, what is man, that thou hast taken thought of him? And the son of man thou hast visited him" (Psalm 8:3-4)?

The Psalmist answers his own question about the importance of people. Remember when the Psalmist use the word "man" in this verse, he means both male and female. He means you and me. The Psalmist wrote his answer, "Yet, thou has made him a little lower than the angels, and hast crown him with glory and honor. Thou hast made him to rule over the works of thy hands; Thou hast put all things under his feet" (Psalm 8:5-6).

"God has made you in his image" (Genesis 2:26). You are just a little lower than the angels. You are special.

Thus God speaks to you, "You are very special to me. I made you. I made you in my image. I love you. I have given you life. Use, enjoy, discover, learn, become the person I made you to be. Keep on becoming the person you can be, living fully and experience my love for you. You are special."

My sister, Sybil Waldrop, tells a story about tadpoles in her book, *Getting Good at Being You* (page 14) which I would like to share with you. She writes, "As a young child, the most delightful and memorable experience I had of God's handiwork was watching tadpoles change into frogs. When I was growing up, my father was pastor of four or five churches at a time. When he preached away from our hometown, we would spend the afternoon with a family who attended the local church. One of my favorite things to do was to find a glass jar and walk along the road in search of a puddle of water where I could find frog eggs—little black balls—each protected by a coat of transparent jelly. Carefully, I would place the jars mouth beneath my wonderful discovery and gather the eggs into the jar. Day by day I would watch as tiny black balls changed into wiggling tadpoles which grew bigger and bigger. A long tail developed and gradually disappeared as frogs formed. Soon tiny amphibious frogs emerged; such was the dramatic transformation. Later I learned the term 'metamorphosis' to describe this change." God and you can work together to bring about a transformation in your life. You can live a fuller life as you make changes in your life which are beneficial to you. If God can change a tadpole into a frog, just think what he can do with you, the highest of his creation.

Cindy is doing very well and enjoying life as never before. Cindy allows the Mary part of her personality to help the Martha part of her to release her anxiety and fear so that she could live a more balanced and enjoyable life.

CHAPTER ELEVEN

CHOOSE WHOM YOU WILL SERVE

I would like to share with you a legend of a shepherd boy. Each day the shepherd boy of our legend would lead his sheep to their food and water. He watched over them, protected them and tended to their every need. As he cared for the sheep, he often picked flowers to give to his mother at the end of the day. One day, as he was leading the sheep to the field, he saw a very beautiful flower on the side of the cliff. When he pulled the flower, a cave door opened before him. He was greatly surprised and a bit frightened, for nothing like this had never happened to him before.

As he cautiously walked into the cave, he looked around. To his amazement, he saw piles of sparkling diamonds, opals, rubies, and other precious stones. He tossed the flower aside and filled his pockets and both hands full of these precious stones. As he started to leave, he heard a voice, "Do not forget the best." The boy thought, "Nothing could be better than these stones." As he walked out of the cave with his hands and pockets full, the cave door closed behind him and the stones turned to dust. You see, he'd forgotten the best. What had opened the cave to the treasure? "The flower." The little boy had forgotten the best! For without the flower, nothing taken from the cave had any value.

The voice in the cave had said, "Do not forget the best," and the challenge of Joshua to the children of Israel was, "Choose you this day whom ye will serve" (Joshua 24). Both these statements call upon us to choose the best, to look for the important, to look for the meaning of life, to set our priorities in order. Our lives and activities are greatly influence and shaped by our thinking. Imedla Shankli, a Unity writer, says, "Your mind is your world. Your thoughts are the tools with which you carve your life's story on the substance of the universe. When you rule your mind, you rule your world. When you choose your thoughts, you choose results . . . Your life is what you think: think straight and your life will become straight for you.

This says to me that where our thoughts are, there is our life. Jesus said, "And a man's foes shall be those of his own household" (Matthew 10:36). Could this mean that the "thoughts" of an individual can be his own greatest foe? The way we think controls our lives. Jesus also said, "and if a house is divided against itself, that house can not stand" (Mark 3:25). Our understanding of God has a tremendous effect upon how we think about life. Jesus said, "The Kingdom of God is within you" (Luke

17:21). I believe that to be true, but there is also the God beyond us. I will not attempt to say what that means to you for that is up to you.

Joshua was a leader of his people, yet he did not command commitment to God for God does not forcibly compel commitment. He exhorts, He calls, but He leaves the choice open. God has left our wills free to choose to reject Him. This liberty is essential to the voluntary commitment of our lives to God. God will not force devotion. The worth of devotion and commitment to God depends on its free willingness to respond.

It is said, "Hope springs eternal in the human breast," but this spark of hope is sometimes reduced to a faint glimmer. Many people cry with Shakespeare's Juliet, "Come weep with me . . . past hope, past help." These people feel trapped in situations and relationships that are destructive which moves from resistance to complete resignation, as they say, "What am I to do? I have no choices!"

(1) The Winds of Circumstance

To all such persons, I would like to say, "As long as you have mental capacity, you have a choice." You may be living with a disease or illness which has or is greatly limiting your life. You may be living in very trying times, faced with problems in your health, your work, in your home and with your finances. You may feel that you are an innocent bystander in a world of conflict of which you feel you have no control. The winds of circumstance do blow and they may not always blow in the way you want to go. Though you cannot regulate the wind, you do have a choice.

Ella Wheeler Wilcox sat by the East River in New York years ago reflecting on the fact that people coming from the same home environment turn out so differently. Inspired by some boats sailing on the river, she wrote, "One ship drives east and the other dives west with the self same winds that blow. 'Tis the set of the sail and not the gales which tells us the way we go." Joshua put it this way, "Choose you this day whom you will serve."

Consider Abraham Lincoln. The winds of circumstance could have blown him into the harbor of mediocrity or ignorance, but he set his sails properly into the gale winds of circumstance. Every gust of wind became for him an opportunity to educate and improve himself until he became a fitting person for the responsibility of sailing the great American ship of state.

You may say, "Hey Chaplain, you are talking about attitudes again." Of course I am, for it is attitude that colors our life. You may object, "But one must be realistic. This situation has happened. It was not my doing, and it is completely beyond my control. I have no choice in the matter and that's just the way things are." I say, "It is not the way things are, it is the way you are seeing them, thinking about them, holding them in your consciousness." Joshua said, "Choose this day whom you will serve." Will you bow before the winds of circumstances or will you choose a new direction in your thinking.

Perhaps you cannot change the facts of the condition in your life, but you do have a choice in how you think about it. You can choose between fear or faith, despair or hope, pessimism or constructive thinking, good or evil, God or something less.

It is often said, "Into each life some rain must fall." Certainly, some rain must fall, for it takes some moisture for growth and the production of fruit even if the rain is not good for a picnic. You can't regulate the weather, but you do have a choice. Someone said, "Experience is not what happens to you it is what you do with what happens to you." We can always choose what attitude we take toward almost anything that comes into our life. We can hate or love, we can resist or run, we can worry about it or we can pray about it. We can accept the difficulty as a crushing defeat or we can make best of it and thus we can go on to renewed effort and achievement.

(2) I Can Think Light

No matter how dark a situation may appear to be, one usually has the choice of turning to the light. The Christophers have a saying, "It is better to light one candle than to curse the darkness." Eric Butterworth tells of a young woman who lost her eyesight. It was the kind of thing that few if any of us would be prepared for. Everyone felt sorry for her. They even felt that the tremendous turmoil of fear and bitterness she was experiencing was justified.

One day something happened to change her thinking and her life. Perhaps she heard the work of Joshua, "Choose you this day whom you will serve." She said, "I may never see light again, but I can think light." She regained a sense of control over her own life for she realized that she did after all have a choice. Now she goes about everything she does with an attitude that is an inspiration to all who know her and it is amazing how many things she had discovered she can do. Everyone has some kind of deficiency in their life, and you can choose to see the light or at least think light.

"Choose you this day whom you will serve." By choosing the best, we can change our negative thoughts to positive thoughts. We can begin to overcome negative thinking by being aware of the negativity in our thinking. Until we are aware of negative thoughts in our mind, we keep acting out of the negativity without realizing why. We can become aware by listening to the words we say to ourselves, "I can't do it. Life is just not fair. I never get a break. If I did not have bad luck, I would have no luck at all. I always get hurt."

(3) The Empty House

Changing negative thinking to positive thinking is more than just saying "No" to the negative. Jesus told a parable about a man who had an evil spirit dwelling in the house his soul (Luke 11:24-27). The evil spirit was causing the man much misery so he decided that if he could get rid of the evil spirit, he could live a productive and happy life. The house of the man's soul was sweep clean and the evil spirit was removed.

An empty house never remains empty. Spiders spin their webs, insects claim the empty rooms, rats run about the house without fear, and dust covers everything. The man cleaned his house of the evil spirit, but he put nothing in its place. Some time later the evil spirit returned to the house of the man's soul. Finding it empty except for the spider webs, insects, rats, and dust, he decided to return and he brought with him seven more evil spirits. The man was then worse off than he was before.

(4) Greek Story of the Sirens

When we get rid of the negative, we must replace it with the positive. The Greeks have a story that may give us some direction. It is about the Sirens who sang so sweetly that sailors could not resist steering toward their island. Many ships were lured upon the rocks and men forgot home, duty, and honor as they flung themselves into the sea to be embraced by the arms which drew them down to death. A man managed to sail his ship safely only if he could resist the Sirens. Finally, they learned a better way to save themselves; they took on board their own better music. When Orpeus sang, who bothered to listen to the Sirens? We must move beyond mere resistance to the negative to say "Yes" to the positive.

Today choose God, good, positive attitudes and then life becomes meaningful. With proper faith, we can choose an attitude toward life that is positive in the face of the good and bad that come to us.

(5) Life Is for Living: Not Quitting

Dr. C. Roy Angell tells the story of a high school track meet held in Alabama some years ago. The athletes were getting ready for the mile race which was one of the big events of the track meet. Since it was expected that the state record for the mile might be broken that day, an unusually large crowd of spectators had gathered at the stadium. One of the schools had a most promising miler. Twice at other events, he had come within seconds of the state record and today he was out to break the record. As they lined up at the starting mark, all eyes were on the tall, good looking young man with a confident, but gracious smile on his face.

On the far end of the starting line was a boy who stood in sharp contrast to the favorite. He was small of stature, his shoulders were bent a little, and one might even wonder why this boy was in the race. The command came to "toe your mark, get set" and then the pistol cracked and the race was on. The favorite easily took the lead. With every lap, he widened the distance between himself and the other runners. The little fellow fell further and further behind. The favorite broke the tape and the state record.

Only a few other runners finished the mile run as most of the runners dropped out as soon as the first three runners crossed the finish line. However, the crowd stood and cheered as the little fellow kept running. Panting, struggling and almost falling, he crossed the finish line. One of the judges ran over to him and handed him a handkerchief. The judge said, "Son, why didn't you stop back yonder when you saw that it was hopeless to win, place or show? Why are you in this race?"

Between gasping, the boy answered, "My school's mile runner got sick two days ago and could not run. The coach wanted a student in every event, so he asked me to run the mile." The judge responded, "You were over a lap behind, why didn't you just quit?" The boy replied, "Judge, the coach didn't send me here to quit, he sent me here to run the mile, and I ran the mile." Though he did not win the race, he was a winner. He chose the best. He was an overcomer and you can be also. You can do it. You can overcome. You can choose the best.

Chapter Twelve
Introducing Hypnosis to Our Congregations and Communities
(A Presentation to the National Association of Clergy Hypnotherapy Convention 1992)

During local seminars, national conventions and discussions with clergy, I often hear the questions, "How does a minister integrate hypnosis into his/her ministry and how does a minister introduce hypnosis to his/her congregation and community?" Though I am a hospital Chaplain and not a local church pastor, I have been thinking about how I would handle this situation if I were the pastor of a local church. (Though this chapter was originally presented to a group of clergy, its contents can be used by non-clergy as well.)

I am aware that there are more misconceptions about hypnosis in our communities than there is knowledge. I understand that some may consider hypnosis as mind control, hocus pocus, or a tool of the devil. Do these misconceptions prevent us from using hypnosis as a valuable tool of pastoral care or do we educate our people about the useful benefit of hypnosis? My response to my own questions is that we educate our people. We teach them that we may use hypnosis for overcoming unwanted habits such as smoking, nail biting, etc; weight reduction and weight control; improved concentration, memory, and study habits; improved athletic ability; overcoming phobia, fears and blocks to a wholesome life, and pain reduction.

Of course the reduction and elimination of pain should not be done at the expense of proper professional medical care. Self-hypnosis may be used when the problem calls for an aspirin or other non-prescription medication, but if the problem persists, one should see a doctor, as pain is an indication that something is wrong and one needs to know what is causing the pain. Hypnosis to relieve pain can be used to augment proper medical care.

One means to introduce your congregation to hypnosis is through your sermons. Though I have references to importance of imagery in a number of sermons, two are more to the point. I share portions of these two with you today.

(1) Body, Mind, Spirit

The first is titled "Body, Mind, Spirit" and the text is Romans 12:1-12 which has the powerful words in the second verse, "But be transformed by the renewing of your mind."

For several years, I have been speaking on what I call "the human trinity." We are all familiar with the Holy Trinity of God, the three in one: Father, Son, Holy Spirit. We humans are also made up of a trinity of our own for we are three in one: Body, Mind and Spirit.

Paul saw this human trinity a long time ago. His understanding of our total being, body, mind, and spirit is demonstrated in the 12th Chapter of the book of Romans. He calls us to total commitment to God which means giving our all: Body, Mind, Spirit. Paul writes, "I urge you, therefore, Bretherm, by the mercy of God, that you present your bodies a living and holy sacrifice to God, which is your spiritual service of worship" (Romans 12:1). Some Christians may have a problem with the verse for some see the body as wicked. The body in their mind is something to be despised and ashamed of. The incarnation of Christ emphasizes the importance of our body. The spiritual worship of which Paul refers is the offering of one's life and all that one does to God.

Paul says that we can offer our body in worship through a change in mind and spirit. "But be transformed by the renewal of your mind" to accept the idea of body, mind, and spirit in unity as being the total person, one can no longer separate life into the sacred and secular. God's command to Moses on Mt. Sinai, "Put off your shoes from your feet, for the place on which you stand is holy ground" did not mean that only that particular piece of ground was holy. God was saying that wherever Moses or you or I may be, that is a holy place for us for God is at that place.

I follow the introduction with illustrations of how we can use the mind and spirit to enhance our life through meditation, prayer, and hypnosis. I conclude with: "When one is functioning in all levels, body, mind, spirit, life is more joyful, more productive and more healthy. We should allow positive thoughts of health, love, trust, faith, righteous living, and confidence to be our first thought in the morning and our last thought before going to sleep at night."

D. Henry Knight Miller states "By faithful reiteration, build into your mind those qualities you desire to express in your life; thoughts of love, health, happiness, success and power. These thoughts are the raw material with which mind, the master builder, the God power within, constructs or reconstructs your life. Give the Builder evil material and the house he builds will be on sand. It will fall. Give the Builder good material and the house not made with hands will withstand all the storms and ravages of time; firm, strong, and unyielding as the Rock of Gibraltar."

(2) Hopeful Expectation

The second sermon is titled "Hopeful Expectation." Romans 15:4-13. Verse 13 reads, "Now may the God of hope fill you with all joy and peace in believing, that you may abound in hope by the power of the Holy Spirit." I began by referring to other messages of hope written by St. Paul. By these and other reference to hope, does Paul mean that we should live our lives in a dream world of wishful thinking? "I wish I had this, I wish I had that." Is that what hope is all about? No! Hope in biblical language is not wishful thinking, but confident expectation of that which is not, but can be. Paul is calling upon us to live our lives in hopeful expectation.

Hope is the outreach of our inner life for courage, meaning, and wholeness. Hope is the reality which transforms mere existence or even self-destructive tendencies to a life lived by positive affirmation. This positive life affirmation is more than giving lip service to hope but it is a way of live. Sometimes our hoping is for something specific while at other times it is more our openness to life's opportunities. In either case, the person of hope lives in a world of open doors and hopeful expectation for the good in life.

It has been said that there are no hopeless situations: there are only people who have grown hopeless about their situation. In the light of experience it is easy for us to despair when things go bad. There are times when we are tempted into a cynical acceptance of a situation and to say, "What is the use?" These are the times when we are tempted to accept a defeated attitude that neither people, nor the world, nor our situation will ever be better. I believe that if we earnestly seek an open door, we can have hope and find meaning in our life. Someone once wrote, "If God shuts one door, He opens another."

We can use hopeful expectation of our physical, emotional, and spiritual improvement and well-being. We are discovering that many of our body's functions which we felt we had no conscious control over can be significantly influenced by our mental attitude. Through relaxation and visual imagery we can learn to control body functions to include the ability to raise or lower temperature and blood pressure, to reduce tension, stress, and pain and to speed up the healing process.

By the use of relaxation, imagery and hopeful expectation, we can have greater affect upon our body and life than we ever thought possible. To follow this procedure you should become as relaxed as possible in either a bed or a chair. When you are comfortable, close your eyes, relax, and let your mind's eyes begin to help you. Imagine the discomfort vanishing, see your illness healed, see your broken bones mended and your wounds healed. As you visualize these things with hopeful expectation, your body begins to respond in a positive helpful way. You are not totally under the control of your distress. Your mind can help you to improve and heal. Visualize or imagine what you want to happen as if it has already happened gives your subconscious mind a model to work toward. It is part of God's healing plan. It will help you experience a better quality of life.

Lew Miller, who was told he would never walk after being wounded in World War II, began to imagine himself, walking, running, driving a car, raising a family, and working. He believed that he would be healed and said, "To believe is to have complete faith in your prayers (thoughts). To believe that you have already received, you need only to visualize yourself as processing it now. Belief in your mental images is the perfect expression of faith."

This hopeful expectation and visualized imagery enhances a person's own immune system which helps you fight germs and infections, decrease tension and stress and helps one alter the stance of helplessness and hopelessness. These methods along with traditional medical treatment and faith in the God who cares can help in healing. Even with those illnesses and injuries which cannot be helped, hopeful expectation brings about an improved quality of life.

The God of hope will cause our hope to grow. The horizons of our hope will expand as God is allowed to be creatively at work within us. In the midst of frustration and conflict there is hope for inner unity and harmony. In the midst of destructive and threatening human relationships, there is the hope for mutually enhancing and fulfilling relationships. In the midst of the pain and wonder of human existence, we live by hope which is based upon faith in God.

Whereas the person of despair lives with a sense of being trapped, the person of hope feels that somehow there is a way out or a way through, and there is the potential for meaning in his or her situation. The person of hope is able to wait, not simply in defeat and resignation, but in anticipation of what is not yet, but can be.

This hopeful expectation can be used not only for health but for every aspect of your life. See what you want to happen in your life not as daydreaming, but as a goal to attain. By doing so, your subconscious has a model to work with. What you think about deeply enough and often enough, you tend to become.

It is extremely important that we allow ourselves to be confronted with the radiant hope of the early church. In the time of the church's beginning, when social, political, and economic condition often seemed intolerable, the people of faith maintained their hope. Radiant with hope, those early Christians talked about hope, sang about hope and lived hope. We can also live in hopeful expectation because of God's love toward us as shown in Jesus Christ. So let us hear St. Paul once more, "Let hope keep you joyful, in trouble stand firm, persist in prayer."

In addition to sermons, you can lead classes for your congregation and community on the positive values of hypnosis to improve life. Jesus said, "I am come that you may have life and have it more abundantly." Hypnosis is one of God's gifts for the more abundant life.

You may want to discuss the use of hypnosis with your church Board of Directors, with women's groups, men's groups, young people's groups and open classes for any one interested.

(3) Presentation to Our Communities

To spread into the community, let other churches and civic clubs such as Rotary, Kiwanis, Lions, etc. know that you are available to speak on the positive uses of hypnosis. You can prepare presentations for time frames of 15 minutes up to an hour and a half.

I share with you a short presentation I use for a civic club meeting. It can be expanded as time allows and can be adopted for a church group presentation. When we hear the word "Hypnosis" we have a mental picture of what hypnosis is. What comes to your mind when you think of hypnosis (give individuals an opportunity to answer). By your answers, it appears that your understanding of hypnosis is based upon the performance of a stage hypnotist or a movie you have seen or a novel you have read. These sources can give you a misunderstanding of hypnosis. Clinical hypnosis is quite different from that of the stage hypnotist or the image of hypnosis as presented in movies or novels.

Hypnosis is really a very common experience which each person goes through from one to many times each day. It is like watching television and becoming so interested in the program, that someone can talk to you, but it just does not register. Has that ever happened to you?

Hypnosis is similar to traveling to a place you have been before, but your mind is on something else and without realizing it, you have passed where you wanted to go. Even though you are not paying attention to where you are geographically, you are driving safely. Your subconscious mind is protecting you, because you are keeping a safe distance between your car and the car in front of you and you are subconscious mind were on automatic pilot. (If time permits, I will give a short history of hypnosis: Genesis 2:21-22, sleep temple, Gasner, Mesmer, etc.)

Your subconscious mind will also protect you in hypnosis for it will not allow you to do anything against your personal or moral convictions. If a suggestion is given that is against your personal or moral convictions, you will either not follow the suggestion if it was a minor thing or you would come out of hypnosis if it was a major concern. Hypnosis is not mind control. You are in control. The hypnotist is only a guide. Some people believe that when you are hypnotized that you are unconscious or asleep, but such is not the case. You will hear everything I say and you will remember much of what I say. Even though I tell each client this, sometimes she/he will say, "I don't think I was hypnotized. I heard every word you said."

(4) Misconceptions

Some other misconceptions are:

1. A person will not come out of the hypnotic trance. *False.* There is not a case in recorded history in which a person failed to come out of hypnosis.
2. A post hypnotic suggestion lasts forever. *False.* A post hypnotic suggestion may not be followed at all or last from a few minutes to a life time.
3. Only weak-minded people can be hypnotized. *False.* The more intelligent and imaginative the person, the easier it is to be hypnotized.
4. Hypnosis is anti-religious. *False.* Hypnosis is neither anti-religious nor pro-religious. It can be good or bad depending on the hypnotist and the client. (If I am speaking to a church group, I expand on this point).
5. A person has to be in a deep trance for hypnosis to be helpful. *False.* People can respond favorable to self-improvement suggestion even in the light state.
6. If you get rid of one symptom by hypnosis, another symptom will take its place. *False.* Symptom replacement rarely ever occurs.

(5) Conscious and Subconscious Mind

How does hypnosis work? Though we have only one mind, our mind is made up of two parts. We have a conscious part which consist of about 10% of our thinking power, and the subconscious part consist of about 90% of our thinking power. Our mind is kind of like an iceberg for only a small portion of the iceberg is above the water (conscious mind) while the great majority of the iceberg is below the surface of the water (subconscious mind).

The conscious mind is a logical, analytical, reasoning, two plus two is four part of mind. The subconscious is not logical. It controls our breathing, pulse rate, blood pressure, heart rate, etc., and it seeks to meet our deepest needs, expectations, and desires and it seeks to continue any habit. The subconscious has two peculiarities which helps us in hypnosis. When the subconscious mind believes something is true, it directs your body to act as if it is true, whether it is or not. The subconscious mind cannot tell the difference between imagination and reality. One day while running, I saw a long crooked object which I perceived to be a snake. My heart beat increased, my breathing changed, and I felt fear. I was ready to run in the other direction when my eyes focused, and I could see it was a stick. So in hypnosis, we use imagery and proper suggestion to help to bring about the wanted changed in a person's life.

Today, I will teach you a self-hypnosis procedure that you can use for improving your life. When practicing self-hypnosis, suggestion should be stated in positive statement instead of negative ones. The subconscious understands positive statement better than negative ones. Repeat the suggestion. The use of visualization and imagination adds to the success of the suggestion by providing the subconscious a model to work with. Do you have any questions?

I usually follow with the hand heavy, hand light suggestion to demonstrate the use of imagination. I then teach a progressive relaxation, self-hypnosis procedure. If time permits, I will do some demonstrations with individual volunteers. Use hypnosis properly and it will lead you to a better life.

Chapter Thirteen
Hypnosis and Religious Faith

(1) Boom Days for Devil Hypnosis

A few years ago, I read an article titled *Boom Days For Devil Hypnosis* by Kathleen Dohney in the *Family Weekly* August 19, 1984 edition. Hearing that title, what ideas, images, thoughts come to your mind? Think about that for a moment and read portions from that article:

The day before she underwent surgery for removal of a facial tumor, Iris Crall made what she thought was an unusual request. "I told my anesthesiologist I needed to be in the right frame of mind and asked if my psychologist could come for a hypnosis session," recalls the 40 year old woman. To Crall's surprise, her anesthesiologist not only agreed but offered to help. The night before the operation Crall was relaxed under hypnosis by her psychologist. The next day, the anesthesiologist used hypnosis to supplement mild general anesthesia.

Crall believes her relaxed positive state of mind, achieved through hypnosis speeded up her recovery. Increasing number of health-care professionals agree that hypnosis can be a great help. Hypnosis is a relaxed state in which the subconscious is more susceptible to suggestion. "Hypnosis can be a great help. Hypnosis is a relaxed state in which the subconscious is more susceptible to suggestion. Hypnosis is a name we give a perfectly normal process," explains Dr. Bernauer Newton. The AMA recognizes a place for hypnosis in medical treatment but the technique has its opponents. "Some conservative religious groups," says Hoffman, "consider hypnosis the work of the devil." When properly administered hypnosis is used in a supporting role in medical treatment, the vote of the health-care community is clear. Hypnosis can help.

Though the article has what I consider a very negative title, it was a very positive article on Hypnosis. The only reference to the devil was in the last paragraph, "Some conservative religious groups consider hypnosis the work of the devil."

Hypnosis is mistakenly viewed as mind control and demonic by many misinformed people. Recently, I received a physician consult to work with a woman for pain management. As I explained the process of relaxation, imagery, and hypnosis, I could see that she was very responsive. She said, "I am really looking forward to the experience, but I need to tell you that my daughter is a self-proclaimed born-again Christian and she may say something negative to you about this. If so, do not pay any attention to her, for I am the one who is hurting and I want to do this."

As I completed the induction, the phone rang. I told the patient, "Just allow the ringing of the phone and my answering it to add to your relaxation." I answered the phone, "This is Mrs. Doe's room. As she is in therapy, please call back in 30 minutes," and hung up the phone.

When the procedure was completed, I walked out of the room and there was her daughter standing in front of the door with arms folded over her chest. She said, "What have you been doing to my mother?" I explained that I had taught her relaxation and self-hypnosis and pain reduction. She responded, "I am a born-again Christian." Before she could continue, I raised my hands and said, "Praise the Lord, so am I." She was speechless, so I continued, "I will bring you some information on hypnosis, but regardless of how you feel about hypnosis, your mother has found it very helpful in the reduction of pain."

Though the title of this chapter is "Hypnosis and Religious Faith," I will be dealing primarily with hypnosis and Judeo-Christian Faith. Whether you are a Christian or not, whether you are religious or not, many of your clients are religiously oriented people. The better you understand the client's religious history, the better you can relate to that person.

(2) Historical Relationships Between Hypnosis and Religious Faith

It could be said that the first written record of the use of hypnosis is found in the Old Testament Book of Genesis 2:21-22, "So the Lord God caused a deep sleep to fall upon man, and while he slept took one of the ribs and closed up its place with flesh, and the rib which God took from man, He made woman and brought her to man." In this incident, God used hypnosis so that Adam felt no pain during the removal of his rib.

Chaplain W. Leo Peacock makes a point with his interpretation of Matthew's account of Joseph's dream concerning taking Mary as his wife. (Matthew 1:20-25) When Joseph discovered that Mary was expecting a child, he decided to break his engagement for he knew the child was not his. The story told of an "angel" or a "messenger" coming to Joseph in a dream. In this dream, the angel told Joseph to take Mary for his wife. Upon waking, Joseph did as the angel suggested. Peacock writes that this a clear description of an individual being given a post-hypnotic suggestion on which he immediately acts on as soon as he comes out of the hypnotic trance.

Paul speaks of being in trance while he was praying in the temple (Acts 22:17). Peter "fell into a trance" and from that experience came to see that God loves all people who come to him (Acts 10:1-48). Though the book of Acts, there are a number of references to the apostles looking into the eyes or gazing into the eyes of a person which resulted in the person being healed (Acts 14:9-10). The practice of "laying on of hands" mentioned in the Bible, used some of the techniques of hypnosis.

Over the centuries, hypnosis has had its ups and downs, but in recent years has become more acceptable. In spite of the successes of hypnosis, we still have those who question its usefulness and others who see it a tool of the devil. One of our missions is to convince those who doubt and enlighten those who oppose, so that people may live better lives.

(3) Religious Organizations' Position on Hypnosis

Hypnosis is neither anti-religious nor pro-religious. It can be used for good or bad depending on the hypnotist and the subject. Today most religious groups accept the proper use of hypnosis. Exceptions among Christian groups are Christian Scientists, Seventh-Day Adventists and some individuals of various churches. In recent years, the Seventh-Day Adventists have lessened their resistance by using relaxation and suggestion therapy. Though many in various churches opposed to hypnosis use the principles of hypnosis (including Christian Scientists and Seven-Day Adventists) in their healing service, they denounce hypnosis.

The Roman Catholic Church has issued statements approving the use of hypnosis. In 1847, a decree from the Sacred Congregation of the Holy Office states, "Having removed all misconception, foretelling of the future, explicit or implicit invocation of the devil, the use of animal magnetism (Hypnosis) is indeed merely an act of making use of physical media that are otherwise licit and hence it is not morally forbidden provided it does not tend toward an illicit end or toward anything depraved."

The late Pope Pius gave his approval of hypnosis. He stated that the use of hypnosis by health care professionals for diagnosis and treatment is permitted. In 1956, in an address from the Vatican on hypnosis in child birth the Pope gives these guidelines: (1) Hypnotism is a serious matter, and not something to be dabbled in. (2) In its scientific use the precautions dictated by both science and morality are to be need. (3) Under the aspect of anaesthesia, it is governed by the same principles as other forms of anaesthesia. This is saying that the rules of good medicine apply to the use of hypnosis.

Except for exceptions noted, no other Protestant Churches have any laws against the use of hypnotherapy. To the best of my knowledge, there has been no opposition to the use of hypnosis in the Jewish Faith when it is used for the benefit of mankind.

Many of the Far Eastern Faiths, including Buddhism, Yoga, Shintoism, and others approve the use of hypnosis and they often use hypnosis techniques in their worship. The Christian Church also uses many hypnotic techniques in their worship. The use of eye fixation on the candles, cross, and pulpit; the bowing of the head and the closing of eyes in prayer.

The Moslem religion has no opposition to hypnosis that I have been able to discover.

For those who oppose hypnosis on religious ground, I remind them of the words of Jon Baptist Van Helmont, "Hypnosis is a universal agent . . . and is a paradox only to those who are disposed to ridicule everything, who ascribe to the influence of Satan all phenomena which they cannot explain."

Some say that hypnosis places the soul in a passively receptive state and opens the door to morbid spiritual influences. If this is correct, then prayer, meditation, the process of going to sleep, and chemical anesthesia place the individual in a similar state to hypnosis. Jesus indicated by his teachings that we should help peoples live life to its fullest and relieve pain whenever possible.

Hypnosis should not be condemned as anti-religious just because a few people misuse it. Some oppose hypnosis because it is used by the occult, but do we condemn prayer because prayer is used by the occult? Hypnosis is a very helpful tool of counseling. Without apology and when appropriate, hypnosis should be used for growth, health, overcoming unwanted habits and the benefit of people.

In the years ahead, may those who discount hypnosis, come to see its value. May those who oppose hypnosis on religious grounds come to view it as a gift of God to help us attain the more abundant life.

Jesus said, "The spirit of the Lord is upon me, because He hath anointed me to teach the gospel to the poor. He hath sent me to heal the brokenhearted, to preach deliverance to the captives and recovery of sight to the blind, to set at liberty them that are bruised" (Luke 4:18). Following this guidance and with the proper use of hypnosis we can heal the brokenhearted, bring deliverance to those in captivity to pain, fear, and phobias; give sight to the emotionally and spiritually blind, and set at liberty those who are bound by unwanted habits. As members of different denominations and religions, let us join hand in brotherhood to share the blessings of hypnosis with others.

Chapter Fourteen
Prayer Therapy

Dr. William A. Parker and Elaine St. John begin their book, *Prayer Can Change Your Life,* "Prayer can change your life anytime, anywhere, at any age. It can heal your diseases, renew your mind and body, calm the storm of daily living from the great tempest of fear and sorrow that threaten to overwhelm, the day by day squalls in human relationship that constantly rock our boat until we view a world distorted by a seasick haze." (p.11)

(1) Dr. Parker and St. John's Study at the University of Redlands

Dr. Parker and Ms. St. John detailed a ten year experiment of Prayer Therapy at the University of Redlands. Their study showed that prayer brought renewal, rebirth, that men and women received "beauty for ashes," and were released from fears, depression, discouragement, and marital difficulties. Dramatic physical healings resulted with stuttering, arthritis, migraine headaches, and high blood pressure as a response to the power of prayer. There were some spectacular recoveries from various diseases, but just as important were the day to day adjustments to life, the "life more abundant," the joy and peace achieved right were they were by individuals who made remarkable adjustments to life.

In their experiments, they had three groups. Group One was the "Psychotherapy" group. They received psychotherapy with no mention of prayer or religion. These people showed a 65% noticeable improvement in both test and symptoms. Group Two was designated, "Random Prayer." These people prayed on their own every night without benefit of psychological insight. They showed no progress in the test, backsliding in some instances. Symptoms were not noticeably improved. Group Three was the "Prayer Therapy" group. The Prayer Therapy group received instructions on positive praying and psychological guidance. The Prayer Therapy group made a 72% improvement in test and improvement of symptoms.

These findings indicate that something was wrong with prayer as understood and practiced by the Random Prayer group. They must somehow have unknowingly prayed amiss for "having asked; received not." The Prayer Therapy group had asked and received. Another result indicated that Prayer Therapy provided something additional to psychotherapy.

(2) Dr. Randy Byrd's Prayer Research

James Wagner in his book, *Ministry of Christ in the Church Today*, writes of another prayer research project that was conducted by cardiologist, Dr. Randy Byrd with a different thrust. In this experiment, the patients were unaware that they were being prayed for by groups recruited by Dr. Byrd. He assigned 393 heart patients, each of whom had been admitted to the coronary unit during a ten-month period, to two groups. Dr. Byrd factored the patients ages and severity of their disease into the division process.

Dr. Byrd then located persons around the country who agreed to pray once a day for each of the 192 patients in the experimental group. Each patient in this group had from five to seven people praying for him or her, but were not told so by the researchers. The second group of 201 patients didn't have individuals from Dr. Byrd's prayer groups praying for them. Dr. Byrd found that the prayed for patients had significantly fewer instances of complication. Only three required antibiotics, compared to sixteen in the other group.

(3) God Hears and Answers Prayer

One of the blessings of faith in God is the assurance that God hears and answers prayer, but at times, we fail to experience that assurance. Could it be that we have no real expectation or confidence that God hears or answers prayer? Perhaps some can identify with the man that associated prayer with playing a slot machine. He said, "It doesn't cost much to play and I might win." That type of experience does not lend itself to a very satisfying prayer life.

As we seek a more meaningful prayer life, maybe we should ask the question "Why pray?" Why teach yourself to pray? Why study to improve your prayer experience? Is it really necessary? Is it an elective in the university of life? Is it a kind of hobby, an optional extra to the main business of being, or should it be an important ingredient of our daily life?

It is my belief that we were created by God to have fellowship with Him. We do not always know what life is all about, but we do know that it exists primarily for relations. A stone is dead, a horse is alive; a stone cannot enter into a relationship with its environment, a horse can. A person can enter into a relationship not only with nature, but also with other people and with God. The richness of our personal life depends upon the quality and depth of our personal relationships. The highest relationship possible is fellowship with God.

In human life, we enter into relationship through fellowship and communication. This is also true of our relationship with God. A person who never prays may know a lot about God—Only the person who prays can know God. This is the strongest reason to pray and the most rewarding. Listen to the Psalmist in 73:25-26, "Whom have I in heaven but Thee? My flesh and heart may fail, but God is the strength of my heart and my portion forever." We pray then in order to enter into, maintain, and deepen our fellowship with God.

(4) One's Image of God

As we accept the need to pray, we see that our image or concept of God greatly affects our understanding of prayer. Dr. William Parker tells of a little boy who was sitting on the floor and drawing on paper. The boy seemed to be so involved in his work that his mother asked, "What are you drawing?" The little boy answered, "I am drawing a picture of God." She responded, "But son, nobody knows what God looks like." The little boy continued to draw and with confidence replied, "Well, they will know what God looks like when I get finished."

Whether we realize it or not, each of us has his or her own image of what God is like in our mind's eye. According to our image of God, we think, we feel, we act, we live and we pray. People see God being: "Not there," "Far away," "Up there," "In the hills from which cometh my help," "In the church," "At the altar," "In the Bible," "Closer than breathing," "Everywhere."

If God is "Not there," then we waste our time to even consider prayer. If God is "Far away," how loud do we have to pray to get God's attention? If God is "Up there," how high do we have to fly in order to communicate with him? If God is "In the hills," what about those of us who live in the low land, such as New Orleans where there is not a hill in sight? If God is only "In the church," do we only get close to him when we go to church? If God is only "At the altar," do we only experience his presence in Holy Communion or at altar calls? If God is only to be found "In the Bible," must we have to have a Bible with us at all times in order to be near God? If God is "Closer than breathing" and "Everywhere," then we can begin to communicate with him wherever we are. Personalizing the statement, "God is everywhere" means "right where I am God is. God is with me." Jesus said "The Kingdom of God is within you." God is here with us "closer than breathing," for the scriptures tells us that God is the friend that sticketh closer than a brother.

Each of us needs to communicate with God in order to reach our fullest potential as a person. Why did Jesus pray? Because he had needs that he could meet in no other way. Why did the disciples pray? For the same reason. As they witnessed the pray life of Jesus, they somehow realized that the deeper needs of their life could be expressed in no other way. It was through prayer that the emptiness of their lives were filled, their faith strengthened, and their hope renewed. Through prayer, they were able to reach their full potential as human beings and so can we.

There is a hymn which speaks to the meaning of prayer. "Lord, what a change within us one short hour spent in your presence will prevail to make, what heavy burden from our bosoms take, what parched grounds refreshed as with a shower! We kneel, and all around us seems to tower, we rise and all the distant and the far, stands forth in sunny outline, brave and clear. We kneel, how weak, we rise, how full of power! Why, therefore, should we do our selves this wrong, or others, that we are not always strong. That we are ever overborne with care, that we should ever weak or heartless be, anxious or troubled when with us is prayer, and joy, and strength, and courage with Thee."

There are times when we do not feel God's presence. What do we do then? During those times when I do not feel God's presence, my prayer goes something like this, "Lord, even though I do not feel you near me at this moment, I accept the fact that you are, so I am going to live my life this day on the basis of your promise to be with me." I have come to discover that in expressing my honest feeling of aloneness that God's presence becomes for me, once again, a reality.

You may be thinking, "I can see the need of prayer, but how do I pray?" As in most of our learning, we learn by doing. You may learn the techniques of playing baseball by studying a book on baseball, but you will never learn to play baseball until you get on the field and make the attempt. This is not to say that the study of theory or techniques is of no value. It is frequently helpful and sometimes essential, but it is not sufficient by itself. Some skills are required almost entirely by practice: typing, playing baseball, driving a car. This is undoubtedly true of the most important way of learning to pray. Prayer is learned in the school of practice.

Prayer may be words, thoughts, or images. Prayer can express feeling of inspiration, devotion, and affirmation. Our prayers are communication with God, but also prayers are closely associated with autosuggestion. Dr. Byrd's experiments show that prayer has elements beyond autosuggestion. Prayers for healing can create an attitude where healing can take place. This is true whether the prayer is for yourself or others.

A prayer I often pray while walking, driving, or just contemplating is, "God's love, joy, peace, and health fills my body, mind, and spirit."

Barbara Von Froggle, a psychology teacher, said that psychologist agree that a person's thoughts affect the body. "We know that the brain releases chemicals. More than two hundred of these are mood-altering. So what you think you do produce in your brain chemically. Taking that medical base, I believe, when you pray, there is a balancing which takes place in the body. You relax, the Holy Spirit has a power of its own that relaxes you and makes you function as God intended."

Our prayer should be affirmations of what we are praying to experience. A lack of affirmations creates a negative attitude which diminishes the effect of one's prayers. The lack of affirmations was a cause for the failure of the Random Prayer Group. "Their form of prayer was negative as well as in complete violation of definite instruction to pray, 'believing ye have you received and ye shall receive.' That promise was fulfilled because as they reiterated their unhappy symptom, holding them directly in the focus of their minds, reaffirming them, then hold them firmly in place. Negative prayer produced negative results."

The Random Prayer group members were often holding their unhappy symptoms directly in the focus of their attention. Over and over they declared they were unhappy, suffering, sinful, and unworthy. As they focused on their problems instead of their solutions, they got what their prayer focused on. They went right on being unhappy, ill, sinful, just as they had been in past. "It is done unto us as we believe." Their words may have requested change, healing, renewal; but their minds focused on their problems.

In our prayers of affirmation, may we learn to see ourselves as we desire to be. As we continue to hold this image in our minds, we re-emphasize it. We tend to experience the images we hold in our mind.

In her book, *How to Manage Stress; Heal Yourself and Be Whole Again,* Lou Coffey-Lewis states that we do not have to shout, demand, or be dramatic in our prayer. Simply ask with childlike faith and trust and your prayers will be answered.

Another element of effective prayer is to pray with the belief that the answer is already there before you even see the evidence of it. Give thanks for the answer before you have experienced it. To give thanks and know without doubt that God has already answered your prayers take a great deal of faith and trust.

Pray as if talking to a close personal friend. Believe that God hears and loves you and let His loving response come to you. God's answer may not always come in the way you expected, but it will come.

When we pray, we must not stop thinking. The mind is the connection link between God and the individual. Prayer should have an element of creative thinking. Emersom said, "Prayer is the contemplation of the facts of life from the highest point of view." Prayer can not help us unless it helps us to change or control our thoughts for as we think in our heart, that is what we are. Change your thoughts and you change your experience.

(5) Guidelines for Effective Prayer (based on Parker and St. John Techniques)

1. Recognize a God of love and meditate on God's love and your relation to him.
2. Understand that God desires healing, wholeness, and abundant life for each person.
3. Release any negative aspects of your life: insecurity, incompetence, anger, guilt, fear, hate, etc.
4. In time of prayer and throughout the day hold positive, healthful, wholesome thoughts and images that are in line with God's love.
5. When praying, believe that you have received the help you have requested and act as if you have received it.
6. In prayer recognize others as in the circle of God's love also and pray for their well-being.
7. Spend time in silence and allow a strong feeling of victory, peace, and serenity to feel your being.
8. Go forth with hopeful expectation.

(6) Binkey's ABC Prayer

It may be helpful to know that God isn't so much concerned with our saying the right things as He is with us saying the real thing. To share with God our feeling and what is on our minds is heard by God just that way no matter how much we may stumble for words to express it. St. Paul in his letter to the Romans (8:26-20) put it this way, "We do not even know how we ought to pray, but through our inarticulate groans the Spirit himself is pleading for us, and God who searches our utmost being knows what the Spirit means."

Dr. R.D. "Sean" Longacre shares this story about his daughter Binkey. This incident occurred when she was just a little girl. Dr. Longacre went to Binkey's room to tell her good night. When he opened the door, she was on her knees by the bed. He heard her praying, "Dear

God, A, B, C, D, E, F . . ." She went throughout the alphabet three times and said, "Amen."

As she got up from her knees, she saw her dad who said, "Binkey, what are you doing?" She replied, "Well you see daddy, I'm not old enough to know all the words yet, so I just keep saying the letters because God will put the words together for me." What a prayer! What Faith!

(7) Luke's Case History

At the request of a patient, I was called to the Emergency Room at Methodist Hospital. I arrived to find a very disturbed man. Luke was a drifter who had taken an overdose of drugs. When I went to his room and introduced myself, he began to cry. With tears running down his face, he said to me, "Why doesn't God love me? I have tried so hard to do what is right, but something always happens to make me go wrong." We talked for awhile about his life and what got him to this point in time. He talked about wanting to experience God's love, presence and peace. He said, "Chaplain, will you pray for me?"

I took his hand and said, "Now just let you eyes closed and begin to relax. In the Psalms, David wrote, 'Be still and know that I am God.' St. Paul wrote to the Romans, 'And in the same way, the Spirit helps us in our weakness; for when we do not know how to pray as we should, the Spirit intercedes for us with groaning to deep for words.' God hears you Luke, even when you do not know what words to say."

(8) The Little Fish in Search of Water

A little fish was swimming near the edge of the river and he heard a teacher speaking to his students. As the teacher and the students were sitting on the banks of the river, the little fish could hear the teacher tell his students, "Water is absolutely necessary for life. Without water, we would perish in a few days." The little fish thought, "If what the man said is true, I better find some of that precious substance called 'water' or I shall die in a few days."

The little fish found other fish and asked them where he could find water, but none of them knew where he could find water. From stream to stream, the frightened fish searched for this life-sustaining water. The little fish found the wisest fish in the river and said, "Please, where can I find the precious substance called 'water' that will give me life." "Waters?" replied the wise fish. "You were conceived and born in water. Water is your environment, water supports your very life. You are surrounded by water!"

You ask, "Where is God?" You are surrounded by God's loving spiritual presence right now. You are conceived in it. You were born in it and your life is sustained by it. You are immersed in God's loving presence. You can now feel his presence all about you as the little fish felt the water all about him.

(9) In the Midst of the Storm

I was quiet for several seconds to give Luke time to let the story of the little fish sink into his subconscious. Now, Luke, use your imagination and put yourself into this story that I'm going to tell you: Now, with your eyes closed let this story of the disciple in the midst of the storm speak to you the message you are ready to hear. Just imagine that you have been with Jesus all day and he has been teaching from the boat because there were so many people there to hear him. Jesus concludes his message and needs a rest so he tells you and the other disciples to sail to the other side. As the boat sets sail for the other side, Jesus lies down and goes to sleep. You and the rest of the company are in no hurry so you decide to do some fishing. It is a terrific day and you have a big catch of fish. All of you are very happy and excited. Meanwhile the gentle waves rock the boat back and forth, back and forth which allow Jesus to sleep soundly.

Almost without warning the sky turns black and the winds begin to blow. The storm winds intensify and the waves rock the boat even harder. Lightening strikes the water near the boat and the boat rocks and tosses as water leaps over the side of the boat. You are afraid that the boat will sink.

As you use your imagination, let that storm on the Sea of Galilee represent any storm that may be going on in your personal life. It may be that you are in the storm of physical pain, of illness, or injury. It could be a financial storm. Do you feel like the disciple? Can you cry out, "Wake up Jesus? Don't you care about us?"

Jesus responded to the cries of the disciples by reassuring them of his presence. "Peace be still, I am with you." When the disciples heard those words, the heart of each disciple began to grow calm. At almost the same time, it was as if the storm was listening for the storm itself became calm.

If you listen now you can hear Jesus say, "Peace be still, I am with you." Peace can come to you with or without a change in your circumstances. In the Bible, the word "peace" never simply means just the absence of trouble or discard. When Jesus comes to us and speaks "Peace be still, I am with you," he is offering the gift of his presence—not just to resolve disharmony, but also to bring us the gift of meaning.

When the cold, black winds of pain, sorrow, illness, injury, financial set backs, or emotion upset blow, there is calm and comfort in the presence of Jesus. When the storm of doubt seeks to uproot the very foundation of faith, there is the presence of Jesus.

No, you are not on the Sea of Galilee, but you feel the winds of the storm and perhaps you are questioning your resources to cope with the situation. The storm in your life may be caused by unrealized dreams, dashed hopes, impairment of health, domestic difficulties, tension on the job, insecurity of position, inadequate finances or conflicts with family or friends.

When the storm of life comes we want to cry out, "Wake up Jesus. Don't you care about us." As we express our need, Jesus comes to us saying, "Peace be still, I am with you," and we experience his presence with us to calm the storm. When the uncertain winds of anxiety blow, there is a steady safety in the presence of Jesus. When the harsh winds of illness or injury blow, there is calm and comfort in the presence of Jesus. When the cold, bleak winds of sorrow and grief blow, there is peace and security in the presence of Jesus. I am not saying that Jesus is a magic cure, but He is with us to either still the storm or help us cope with the storm. To experience the presence of Jesus is to experience peace in the midst of the storm. May you experience that peace today. "In Jesus name, Amen."

With the "Amen," he thanked me and said, "Do you want to know what meant most to me?" I responded, "Yes, please tell me." He said, "You touched me."

I saw Luke the next day before he was discharged and he looked like a different person. He said, "That was an unusual prayer you prayed yesterday. I don't remember ever hearing a prayer like that before. You made me a part of the prayer. I was living the prayer. It seemed like I was in the boat with Jesus during the storm. Thank goodness Jesus woke up and said, "peace be still." How is Luke doing now? I don't know for I have not seen him since his discharge from Methodist Hospital.

(10) Mahatma Gandhi's Prayer

I conclude this chapter with a story about Mahatma Gandhi who lead India to independence. Louis Fischer, who was Gandhi's friend and biographer, wrote of visiting Gandhi. He writes that he saw only one decoration on the mud walls of his hut; a black and white print of a painting of Jesus with the inscription, "He is our peace." Mr. Fischer asked Gandhi about it and he responded, "I am a Christian, and a Hindu, and a Moslem, and a

Jew." This is a parable of God's love and even though it may be difficult to attain, may we never be too narrow to admire it when it flashes across our horizons. Gandhi once wrote, "In the midst of death, life persists; in the midst of untruth, truth persists; in the midst of darkness, light persists; hence I gather that God is life, truth, and love. He is love. He is the supreme Good."

Chapter Fifteen
Stress Management

In my book, *Human Trinity Hypnotherapy* I discussed the harmful effects of the improper handling of stress. Because I believe it is an important issue, I am including a second look at stress and how we handle stress to reduce its destructive force in our lives and the lives of others. In the order of medical statistics, heart failure is the number one cause of human death; cancer, number two; stroke, number three; accidents, number four; and suicide, number five. The first three listed may be called organic causes of death, while number four is partial psychological and number five is totally psychological. Behind all of these, the cause of much of our illnesses and injuries is the improper handling of stress.

Behind the mask many people put on for the public, many are disturbed, many are perturbed, others are worried to the point of confusion, and some are just frustrated with life as it is. Many do not feel up to par; they have a tiredness, a pain, a disagreeable feeling, an inner hurting. They are worried about many things and are experiencing apprehension, fears, and irritations. They are missing all to much of the good life. They have traveled through the years trying to avoid but always managing to experience new troubles and negative feelings. They are irritated more than happy; tensed more often than calm.

They come to the physician because of their physical symptoms rather than the strain of their inappropriate handling of stress which may be the cause of their problems. In most cases, they are unaware that their physical symptoms are a reflection of their reaction to stress. They don't like the tiredness, the pain, the symptoms and they want to do something about them. They are amazed when told that the most effective way to deal with the symptoms is to live differently. They have to learn how to handle emotional stress and make healthy life-style changes in how they react to life.

The human body was designed to resist disease, but the improper handling of stress, weakens our natural fortification against disease. It is my assumption and it is supported by many in the medical field that stress plays a part in most of our illnesses and injuries.

Stress is a part of life and it can be helpful or harmful to us. Stress can motivate us to be successful in life and to improve our life style habits. On the other hand, stress can weaken our resistance to illness and can be a destructive force in our lives. As stress cannot be found outside an individual, therefore it becomes obvious that it has to be dealt with from within.

Arthur Gordon tells the story of knowing an old psychiatrist named Smiley Blanton. Smiley was famous for a book he had written titled, *Love or Parish,* and he believed that title to be literally true. Since Gordon and Blanton were from the same area of the South, they enjoyed tall tales and legends from the region.

"Down in Georgia," Gordon once told Smiley, "Some folks say that if you cage a mockingbird, another mockingbird will come along and feed the prisoner a poisoned berry to put it out of its misery. Do you believe that?" Smiley replied, "Well, no, but I must say I have a lot of patients who keep feeding themselves poisoned berries; anger, hatred, jealously, self-doubt, and self-pity. They keep these poisons locked up inside of them and then wonder why they are sick."

"Can you usually help them?" Gordon asked. "Sometimes, sometimes not. The most difficult are the ones who tell me frantically that they've tried everything possible to solve their difficulty and nothing works and so assume nothing can work. Sometimes, I say to them, stop trying. There are great currents of love and healing flowing through this universe, but you're blocking them with all this gloom and despair. Go home, stay calm, do nothing for awhile. Get out of your way, Get out of God's way. Then wait and listen."Gordon asked, "and does that work?" Smiley responded, "More often than you think. Then they go around saying I cured them. But, you know better than that and so do I."

Dr. Irving Oyle states that the images of a disease must first be in the mind before it materializes into the body. Before health can return, Oyle believes that a person's thinking patterns must change. Thoughts are living vibrations. It has been proven that thoughts actually produce electrical impulses in the brain and that these impulses go throughout the body to produce actual physiological changes in the body moment to moment. Angry and hateful thoughts produce physiological changes that can be measured. During demonstrations of biofeedback machines, in which an individual was told to think negative, angry, thoughts, changes took place. Devices on the machine registered physiological data such as muscle tension, increased muscle relaxation, decreased heat and pulse rate, and change the skin temperature. The way one thinks does affect one's body for good or bad.

Coffey-Lewis adds that the best and most important step in using your own thinking for healing is to recognize that you choose what you want to think. No person, no condition, has any power over your thoughts unless you allow it to happen. You can choose to decide to take responsibility for your thoughts. You can choose to be happy and joyful. By allowing negative thought and worry to overtake you, you are also choosing. You can create your own world however you want it with your thoughts. This does not meant that thoughts alone can cause disease, but improper thinking does play a role in many diseases, including ulcers, chronic back problems, headaches, and even cancer. Blair Justice states that many of our sicknesses are strongly influenced, both in its beginning and duration, "by the way we think and behave—demanding no frustration, seeing problems as overwhelming, looking for the worst, alienating ourselves and others, smoking, overdrinking, overeating, not exercising." Blair goes on to say that "If a person has poor coping skills, deficient social support and high stress, then the internal balance of your bodies may be easily upset and your resistance lowered."

Louis Orton states that worry puts a strain on an individual mentally and physically. Worry interferes with the flow of digestive juices and affects the digestive system. Worry alters the chemical composition of blood and lymph. The continued effect of worry on the body can "provide a suitable ground for more serious diseases."

An A.P. Science reporter writes that a healthy outlook helps heal the heart and that a pessimistic attitude is a killer. Dr. Daniel Mark said, "Optimism is a good thing. When people give up and feel they are not going to make it, it's usually a self-fulfilling prophecy." In a follow up of 1,719 men who underwent heart catheterization, 14% said they doubted that they would recover enough to resume their daily routine. After one year, 12% of those who were pessimistic had died compared with 5% of those who were optimistic about getting better. Feelings of sadness, depression, hostility, being unmarried and having no one at home to talk to seemed to contribute to more deaths.

As early as 1914, Dr. Walter Cannon began describing how the refusal to deal with anger and fear can trigger physical illnesses. When anger and fear go unchecked, they can trigger many physical illnesses. You may be thinking it is germs and other factors rather than feelings such as worry, anger, and guilt that causes sickness. I am not saying that stress alone causes illness, but that it can have an effect upon our resistance.

Studies have shown that identical twins with the same genetic tendency toward a given illness, or two people with similar germs within them, or two people who breath the same polluted air, one might get sick while the other will not. The one who gets sick is generally the one who is having difficulty with emotionally stressful situations such as overworked, worry, anger, guilt, and fear. By being able to identify and work through these problems, we can reduce the chance of being ill.

David Hilton, M.D., is convinced that the most important dimension to health is the spiritual. Even in the midst of poverty some people stay well, while among the world's affluent many are chronically ill. Why? Medical science is beginning to affirm one's beliefs and feelings are the ultimate tools and power for healing. Unresolved guilt, anger, resentment, and meaningless are found to be the greatest suppressors of the body's powerful, health-controlling immunity system, while loving relationships are among the strongest augmenters. Those in harmony with the Creator, the earth, and their neighbors not only survive tragedy and suffering best, but grown stronger in the process.

There is a connection between illness and injuries and such things as loneliness, hopelessness, fear, resentment, joylessness, stress and lack of meaning. Our feelings about ourselves and others and the quality of our relationships have more to do with how often we get sick and how soon we get well than do our genes, chemistry, diet, germs, or environment. Accepting this view, we realize that we play a part in our health for good or bad. This is not said to cause guilt for being ill, but provide hope for better health.

An interesting and unusual experiment was conducted at the University of Wichita. It was under the direction of Dr. N.H. Panko, head of the Department of Psychology. A graduate student, Fred J. Snyder, wore a pair of special inverted vision glasses for a month to test his reactions. During this period, Fred lived in an upside down and backward world. Right became left, up became down. When he ate, it seemed as if he were suspended from the ceiling and his food was hanging on his plate defying gravity. When he reads a book, he reads it bottom to top and right to left. Everything was upside and backward.

Ours is a topsy-turvy world and we do not need up side down glasses to lose our perspective and bearing. Confusion has become normal, trouble is all about us. Violence has become a way of life for many. Values are misplaced and proper direction seems to have been lost. With these problems, we have a tendency to translate these stress factors into body symptoms.

(1) Body Syndromes

The theory of body syndromes as described by Dr. John Kappas in his book, *Professional Hypnosis Manual,* is based upon the principle that whenever an emotional trauma is present, a corresponding physical reaction will take place. Dr. Kappas states that these physical reactions, called "Body Syndromes," will in turn reflect the cause of the emotional problem according to the area or areas of the body that becomes affected by the pain, pressure, or tension. Dr. Kappas' five syndromes are:

1. The *Crying Syndrome* involves the area of the body covering the chest, head and back of neck. The cause of the *Crying Syndrome* is the inability to make a decision, either because it is predicated on someone else's action, or because of an inability to make decisions due to past conditioning. Headaches are the most common characteristic of the *Crying Syndrome.* Because of frustrations from indecision, the brain signals the muscles in the scalp to tighten, causing pain. Sometimes the tightening becomes too severe, and it constricts the blood vessel in the head, resulting in migraine headaches. Some of the other easily recognizable symptoms of the *Crying Syndrome* are: crystallization of the eyes or problems with tear ducts, causing the eyes to water; sinus congestion; constriction of throat muscles; gastric pressures in the chest area; tightening of muscles in the back of the neck; canker sores in the mouth; tightening of jaw muscles or grinding of teeth. Each one of those physical reactions can be associated with an emotional or mental cause. For instance, the head pressures represent inability to make the decision; watering eyes and sinus congestion symbolize not wanting to see the situation that is causing the indecision; constriction in the throat, tightening of jaw muscles, or grinding of teeth result from not wanting to express anything about the area of indecisiveness. If improperly handled or not handled at all, indecisiveness moves into frustration, and from there to melancholy, depression, and finally futility. Chronic indecisiveness can be classed as a major problem in today's fast moving society.

2. The bodily areas affected by the *Responsibility Syndrome* are the shoulder, the upper back, and the upper spinal area. The psychological causes are too much responsibility, fear of the weight of responsibility, or neglecting, not accepting, or not facing responsibility. The psychological reaction of the *Responsibility Syndrome* is tightening of the back and shoulder muscles. In some instances, if excessive or rapid movement or lifting is attempted when these tensions are present, physical damage can be done to the back.

3. The *Sexual Frustration, or Guilt Syndrome:* The areas of the body affected by *Sexual Frustration, or Guilt Syndrome* are the stomach, groin, and lower back. The psychological causes can be sexual frustration, religion-linked sexual

guilt, guilt about infidelity, feelings of sexual inadequacy, and so forth. The physical symptoms can be stomach cramps, constipation, acid stomach, excessive menstrual cramps with too much bleeding or no bleeding at all, vaginal or bladder infections, prostate or testicle pain, and kidney problems.

4. The *Fight or Reaching Syndrome:* The areas affected by the *Fight or Reaching Syndrome* are the arms, hands, and fingers. The psychological symptoms involve the need to express, with denial or suppression of that need; the inability to reach for something one desires because of lack of feelings of self worth; and a feeling of deep rejection as a result of reaching for unattainable goals. The physiological effects are warts or little blisters on the hands or fingers, tightening of the joints and muscles in the hands, or extremely hot or cold hands. Arthritis and rheumatism are related problems.
5. The *Flight Syndrome* affects the area from the thighs to the feet. It indicates a need to run or escape (emotionally or physically) from a particular situation or involvement. The psychological causes are a fear of facing certain situations because they may be painful. Other causes are boredom, fear of disaster, and fear of success. The physiological symptoms are blistering between the toes or on the bottom of the feet, cold feet because of poor circulation, and leg pains.

A person may be affected by one or more of the syndromes described above at any given time. For example, a headache and tight back muscles in combination indicate an inability to make decisions about responsibility. Tension in the back muscles and pain in the legs denote the responsibility is causing a person to want to escape from a situation that he cannot actually leave. In my opinion, most physical ailments are caused by body syndromes that remain too long without proper treatment.

(2) Some Things You Can Do to Reduce Stress

1. *Exercise:* Recall that your body often manifests the "fight or flight" response to stress. The body is prepared for strenuous effort. Regular physical exercise will help you to use the extra sugars and fats in your blood caused by stress. If you

are angry, try to blow off steam physically by activities that are helpful to you. I like to walk a couple of miles a day which helps me to reduce stress. For others, it may be various sports, running, working at your hobby, or just taking a walk. Of course, before beginning any strenuous activities, you should see your doctor.

2. *Balance work and recreation:* Schedule time for recreation. Learn to play and have a good time. All work and no play can make you a nervous wreck.
3. *Learn to accept what you can not change:* To accept does not meant to like. It means to do the best you can under the circumstances.
4. *Talk out your worries:* It helps to share worries with someone you trust, such as a friend, family member, clergy person, teacher, professional counselor, or some other trusted person.
5. *Avoid self medication:* Although there are many chemicals such as alcohol or drugs which can mask your symptoms, they do not help you adjust to stress.
6. *Get enough sleep and rest:* Lack of sleep can reduce your ability to deal with stress.
7. *Prayer and Meditation:* Life is more than just being alive mentally and physically. To be the whole person that we were meant to by our Creator, we have to be alive spiritually as well as physically and mentally.
8. *Learn to relax* and use your mind, progressive relaxation and self-hypnosis to help you deal with stress.

(3) Katie's Case History

Katie was a 50-year-old female, married with a 20-year-old son who lived at home. Katie saw me once a week for two weeks and every other week for several months. Her presenting problem was allergies which were intensified with current stressful situation at home. Katie and her husband were friendly but there was little affection between the two which was a problem for her. Her son was without a job and that was also a concern.

She said that her allergies went back at least to her high school years and she had frequent headaches. She tested 50/50 on the suggestibility questionnaire and the suggestibility exercises. She responded equally well to direct and indirect suggestions. From the "Taste the lemon" exercise, I determined that she was a visual person with facial response which indicated that she could almost taste the lemon. I converted a "Heavy hand, light hand" suggestibility exercise into an induction.

After a progressive relaxation exercise, I lead her through the "Walk in Country: Backpack" imagery which will be recorded in the weight control case history. The suggestion was that if she was ready to be released from the conscious and subconscious need for her allergies, her first finger of her right hand would rise. The finger rose with a jerky motion and remained up until I suggested that it go down to her lap.

(4) Overcoming Allergies

The word, "allergy" pertains to a condition or sensitivity to some substances, called, "allergens." It can be emotionally induced or intensified by stress.

A person who is allergic reacts in a way different from the way others react when they eat, inhale, or touch the allergen . . . Allergy is actually a normal reaction of the body. However, there are times when it is being misused by the body . . . I'll explain what I mean by that . . . If a person inhales a harmful irritant or bacterial toxin, it is normal for a watery secretion to come out of the nose . . . That's the way the body reacts to cleanse the harmful irritant or bacterial toxin out of the body to keep the body in its normal, healthy condition.

That is a normal reaction, a natural allergy . . . But it is abnormal and can be very distressing for a person's nose runs just because he or she gets near fresh cut grass, or near a dog, or near a cat. The reason some people become allergic and others don't has been a mystery for many years. The medical profession has been baffled as to the reason some people develop a runny nose because of rag weed . . . mold . . . dust . . . or other triggers; while others are not bothered by any of these things.

In recent years many studies have revealed that thoughts or ideas in a person's mind can cause allergic condition to develop. By saying that thoughts or ideas cause allergic conditions to develop does not mean that the person wants to have those allergic reactions. People do not want to have hay fever, runny noses, or other allergic symptoms . . . It is misunderstandings in the subconscious level of the mind that causes those condition to develop.

Tension and stress have also been found to contribute to allergic reactions. Emotional factors, anxiety, or even grief are often found to be the cause of these conditions.

In most cases involving allergic conditions, it has been found that the situation or circumstance caused the condition has changed, but the person continues to have the allergy because it has become a learned reaction of the mind. In other words, the subconscious mind caused the allergic condition to continue merely because it has become a habit. However, anything the mind has caused, the mind can also cure . . .

Your subconscious mind is understanding what I've been telling you, and is causing all of your body processes to function properly and to cleanse all impurities out of your body and eliminate the allergic symptoms you have been experiencing. You're noticing changes in your life, because your mind is releasing those ideas, thoughts, imprints and impressions that caused the allergies to develop. The usual pattern of being allergic is progressively decreasing . . . Beginning right now, your subconscious mind is understanding that you want to get rid of all unnatural allergies. Allergies are progressively having less and less control over you . . .

In going through various experiences during your normal, everyday living, your subconscious mind receives information that caused you to develop the habit of allergies, but your subconscious mind is understanding that the information was misunderstood, and you can see it from a more knowledgeable, more mature point of view, and you want it changed and corrected. You want the processes of your body to function properly and cleans all impurities and substances which have any allergic effect eliminated from your body through the natural process of your elimination system . . .

Your subconscious mind is causing you to become desensitized to all substances and conditions which, in the past, have caused you to suffer abnormal allergic reactions . . . You desire to be released from the harmful effect of these allergies, and your subconscious is getting rid of the habit of responding to situations and conditions that has been causing you to experience allergies . . . You are continuing to relax more and more, and your subconscious mind is accepting these suggestions, and is improving your health, and enabling you to live life in a more peaceful, more calm, more relaxed way . . . Each day these suggestions become more effective . . . You are learning to use these principles of relaxation which you are now experiencing in all phases of your daily life, and that keeps you calm and relaxed during your daily life.

In every situation or circumstance that comes up in your life, you are calm and relaxed. Your nerves are relaxed and steady, and you'll be able to do things in a relaxed way. You are able to cope with your everyday changing circumstances in a peaceful way. Regardless of what comes up in your life, you are in control of your emotions and feelings. That causes the allergic reaction to keep fading away more and more, and soon is gone completely.

Over the next few weeks, Katie reported feeling better with fewer allergic attacks occurring. We did an age regression and she went back to age five. However, she opened her eyes and said, "I am not ready for this now." I said, "OK, just let the scene fade out and relax even deeper. Relaxing more and more with each breath you take." To close out that session, I used "Therapy Between sessions."

(5) Therapy Between Sessions

After you come out of this hypnotic state, you can continue reviewing, examining, and exploring the storehouse of your subconscious mind and work out solutions to these problems in a way that is pleasing to you. If it is important for you to consciously be aware of the situation you were not ready to deal with, you will remember. When you are ready, you are able to look at it with me or another professional. As you go about your daily activities and during your sleep, your mind can be assessing information that is contained in your subconscious mind. You can understand that information from a completely different point of view than when the information went into your mind . . . You can work out the solution now from a more knowledgeable, more mature point of view.

After you come out of this hypnotic state, your subconscious mind can continue reviewing all imprints, impressions, thoughts, ideas, and other information that has gone into your mind and had anything to do with causing this problem . . . Your mind can begin to work out a pleasant solution to this problem in a way that helps you overcome the problem.

In the past you may have had some doubts, but those doubts are leaving, and all those doubts are soon gone completely . . . Those doubts are being replaced with a strong sense of confidence and sureness . . . We are having these sessions because you are determined to overcome this problems . . . It has controlled your way of life long enough and you are determined to be released from its control . . . Your subconscious mind is now working for you to overcome this problem in a way that is pleasing and acceptable to your conscious mind . . . You begin to notice pleasant changes taking place in your life as your subconscious mind works out a very pleasant solution to this problem . . .

(You can use "Therapy Between Sessions" when subconscious questioning reveals that the subconscious is not ready to give up the problem or when the client is unable to deal with the problem during the session or is unable to release all negative feeling and causes of the problems when using "Waterfall For Cleansing," "Hand to Face for Therapy" or other releasing techniques.) During the next session, I used "Hand to Face for Therapy" with Katie.

(6) Hand to Face for Therapy

In a moment I'm going to ask you to open your eyes and put your (right or left) hand up in front of your face with the palm of your hand toward you, and you are able to look at your fingers and the palm of your hand. As I talk to you, you continue experiencing a more soothing and peaceful relaxation coming over your whole body.

Open your eyes now and lift your hand up a little above eye level and press your fingers tightly together. You become aware of all the feelings and sensations in your fingers and hand, and you keep experiencing a more peaceful, soothing sensation coming over your whole body. It keeps becoming easier for you to respond to the suggestions I tell you.

You notice the feelings and sensations in your fingers and your hand, and your fingers feel like they want to start spreading apart. Don't try to make them spread apart deliberately, and don't try to keep them from spreading apart. They spread apart all by themselves, easily and gently. And as your fingers are spreading apart, you notice that your eyes start feeling heavy, and your eyes keep feeling heavier and heavier. And your eyes feel like they want to close as you drift into a calm, peaceful, deepening, hypnotic state of relaxation.

You experience a soothing drowsiness coming over your entire body, and your eyes are closing gently . . . Your eyes are soon closed . . . It keeps becoming less and less important for your eyes to be open, and by the time your eyes close, you are in a deep, calm, very peaceful hypnotic state. Notice that your fingers want to spread apart, and you are letting the natural feelings happen. As your fingers are spreading apart you can notice that your eyes keep feeling heavier . . . Being hypnotized is always a very pleasant, calm, soothing, very enjoyable, restful experience (pause). (Note: After fingers have started spreading and eyes have closed, continue as follows.) In a moment, your (right-left) hand and arm begin moving toward your face, and you keep drifting into an even deeper hypnotic state . . . Your hand and arm move toward your face, but your subconscious mind does not permit your hand to touch your face until your mind has worked out a solution to that problem.

You have been experiencing that problem for some time now, and consciously you haven't been able to resolve it. I don't know what has been causing that problem, but the subconscious part of your mind does have the information . . . so your subconscious mind can review, examine, and explore the information in your mind and find out what has been causing that problem.

Your subconscious mind can review all the imprints, all the impressions, all the thoughts and ideas in your mind that have been causing that problem . . . and your mind can assess, evaluate, and understand that information now from a more knowledgeable, more relaxed, more calm, more mature point of view . . . and can work out a solution and resolve that problem rapidly and completely. Your subconscious mind is reviewing that information thoroughly and understanding that it is OK to resolve that problem for now and forever . . . and when your mind has resolved that problem, then your mind causes your hand to touch your face.

You are continuing to move into a deeper, more peaceful, more detached state. It feels good to keep relating more. Your mind is cooperating. Reviewing that information, working out a very pleasant solution to that problem . . . and you are easily and gently moving into a more comfortable state of relaxation . . . Your subconscious mind is hearing every word I say and is working out a pleasant solution without any conscious effort by you . . . Your fingers have spread apart, and your subconscious mind is causing your hand to move toward your face, but your hand does not touch your face until your subconscious mind understands the causes and effects of what has been causing that problem and knows that it is OK for that problem to be resolved completely . . . When your mind knows it is OK for that problem to be resolved then your hand touches your face as a signal that the problem has been resolved . . . and you really are pleased . . .

You are in a very deep, very calm, comfortable state now . . . By permitting your mind and body to relax through your own ability to concentrate on the words I say, you notice later, after you come out of the hypnotic state, that you feel much better mentally and physically . . .

You're doing good . . . It feels good to continue relaxing . . . and later, when you come out of the hypnotic state your whole body feels good from the top of your head all the way down to the bottom of your feet . . . Your hands, arms, and shoulders are relaxed and comfortable . . . and you are confident and happy . . .

Your subconscious mind is very sensitive to everything I say, and is hearing and receiving the suggestion I'm telling you . . . Causing each suggestion to begin working immediately and continue working automatically as you go about your daily activities, and you experience many wonderful benefits from being in this comfortable, relaxed state of hypnosis . . .

You are aware that your own subconscious mind is working out the solution to that problem . . . Your subconscious mind knows what to do . . . and is doing it in just the right way to resolve the problem completely . . . Some of those experiences your mind is reviewing may not seem to make sense . . . yet quite often those are the ones that have the most meaningful effect in solving the problem. Past experiences that have been misunderstood subconsciously can now be understood from a different point of view and your mind is able to work out the solution to that problem in ways you do not consciously understand . . . So your subconscious mind is causing your hand and arm to continue moving toward your face to indicate that it is reviewing, examining and exploring the information that has been causing that problem and is working out the solution . . . You already have all the ingredients, all the capabilities, all the skills that you need, and all the knowledge that you need to overcome this problem. (Continue on if hand has not touched face.)

Right now it may seem like you are experiencing some kind of a dilemma . . . You may not be consciously aware of what needs to be done to work out the solution of that problem, but that's one of the amazing wonderful things about your subconscious mind . . . because, even though you do not consciously know what to do, your subconscious mind has all the knowledge it needs to work out the solution in a very pleasant way . . . and your subconscious mind is bringing that important information forward now, and is resolving that problem for now and forever . . . Consciously you have decided that you want to overcome this problem and you have the right to make that decision . . .

In the past there was something keeping that problem from being resolved . . . Whatever it was that has been causing that problem is soon to be changed . . . Your subconscious mind is understanding it from a more knowledgeable, more mature point of view, and knows that it is OK for that problem to be resolved completely and permanently . . .

That decision has got to come from you . . . and from your own mind . . . There is no need for it to come from me . . . because it is only when your mind makes that decision that the problem is resolved . . . You know that your mind is the only part of you that can cause the changes that are needed to resolve that problem . . . And your mind can cause those changes as you go about the activities of your daily life.

Your subconscious mind keeps your heart pumping the blood through your circulatory system, keeps you breathing, enables your digestive system to continue functioning properly, enables you to talk when you decide to talk, walk when you decide to walk, and has been doing thousands of other things that your conscious mind has not been consciously aware of . . . The importance of all this is realizing that you can trust your own subconscious mind to take care of you . . . You can be sure your own mind is causing you to experience pleasant changes that are needed to resolve that problem.

You can trust your own mind to do what is needed to overcome that problem and all other problems when given proper guidance . . . and that's what you are doing now . . . Your mind is receiving the proper guidance needed to work out the solution . . . and you are noticing the pleasant changes taking place . . . (her hand touches her face and a deep sigh was followed by a very pleasant expression on her face. If her hand had not touched her face, I would have continued with "Therapy Between Sessions") I continued: You are responding properly . . . Your subconscious mind is doing what is needed to resolve that problem . . . You can be pleasantly surprised to find that your subconscious mind causes this to happen in an easy, natural way . . . It gives you a lot of satisfaction to know that your own mind is working out the solution to that problem and your goals can be accomplished satisfactorily . . .

In another session, Katie said she was better able to deal with anger, take life more easily, was less attentive to details, and has come to an understanding that she can't change everyone around her. In the hypnotic state, I continued . . .

(7) You Can Let Go of the Garbage

A group in New York City once advertised that they were taking reservations for a trip to the moon. Prospective travelers were warned that the moon was a cold and arid place where movement would be difficult and conversation without radio transmission would be impossible. In spite of these drawbacks, over 18,000 people requested reservations.

Those making reservations were asked to explain why they wanted to go to the moon. There were a number of reasons given, but two reasons emerged as leaders. Many stated that they wanted to go because of the adventure involved, but most wanted to escape the earth and their own problems. Remember the man who went to the other side of the world to get away from his problems only to find that he had brought his biggest problem with him—himself.

You don't need to run away from your problem, but to use your mind to help you overcome or endure your problem in a constructive way. You can do this by a change in your attitude from defeat to hope and meaning.

You are carrying a lot of baggage which you can get rid of. A woman with a heavy suitcase boarded a bus. Once on the bus, she continued to hold her baggage. The driver said to her, "You can put your baggage down, lady, the bus will carry it for you." You can let it go.

Suppose we tried to keep our garbage in our homes, hiding the scraps and litter away in various parts of the house, day after day and week after week. Think of the smell and disease that would poison the entire household. The simple principle holds true in our emotional life as well. If we let the garbage of life keep piling up inside us, it eventually works us harm. Let the garbage go. Feel good about yourself. As you do, your self-confidence increases and you grow emotionally and spiritually. You can change your mind and change your life. St. Paul wrote in Colossians 3:8-10, "But now you also put them all aside: anger, wrath, malice, slander, and abusive speech from your mouth . . . since you laid aside the old self . . . and have put on the new self who is being renewed to a true knowledge according to the image of the one who created him."

Close to the end of her therapy, Katie asked to be regressed as she felt that she was ready for it. She went back to being a baby in her mother's arms. As her mother was crying over the absence of her husband who was fighting in the war, baby Katie wanted to cry but could not. This was the Initial Sensitizing Event (ISE).

She then went forward in her regression to her Godfather's death. She loved him very much. On the night of his wake, she stayed at the house of a friend and had lots of fun for which she felt guilty. She did not cry at the funeral. This occurred at the age of five and was the Symptom Producing Event (SPE). Following that she would occasionally have an allergic reaction which intensified during her high school years. She then recalled several events when she wanted to cry, but couldn't. These were the Symptom Intensifying Events (SIE).

During these sessions, Katie's spiritual life had changed and she was experiencing a real closeness to God. I concluded our last hypnotic session with the story of the Velveteen Rabbit.

(8) The Velveteen Rabbit

Margery Williams wrote a child's story which presents a great truth about real life. The Velveteen Rabbit is the story about a rabbit who was made of velveteen and stuffed with sawdust. The rabbit felt insignificant among the other fancier toys of the boy's nursery. His best friend was Skin Horse who had lived in the nursery longer than any other toy.

"What is real?" The rabbit asked Skin Horse, "Does it mean having things that buzz inside you and a stick-out handle?" Skin Horse responded, "Real life isn't how you are made, it's something that happens to you. When a child loves you for a long time . . . really loves you, then you become real."

The rabbit continued his questioning, "Does it happen all at once, like being wound up, or bit by bit?" The Skin Horse answered, "It doesn't happen all at once. You become, it takes a long time . . . generally by the time you are real, most of your hair has been loved off, your eyes have dropped off, and you get very loose in the joints and very shabby. But these things don't matter at all, because once you are real you can't be ugly, except to people who don't understand."

In time the rabbit became real. He knew it one day when he had been left in the yard after a day of play with the little boy. Nana, the nurse, had to bring the rabbit to the boy before he would go to sleep. As she handed the rabbit to the boy, Nana said, "Fancy, all that fuss for a toy." The boy took the rabbit and responded, "Give me my bunny. You mustn't say that, he isn't a toy, he's real." When the rabbit heard that, he was overjoyed because he was real at last. He was no longer a toy, he was real. The boy himself had said it. God says to you that you are not play things of fate, you are real and as such, you can experience life more abundantly. Because God loves you, you receive the gift of life and begin the process of real life.

(9) Stress Bibliography

Blair, J. (1987). *Who Gets Sick.* Peak Press. Houston, Texas

Crowe, C. (1952). *On Living With Yourself.* Abington Press, Nashville, TN.

Hay, L. (1984). *You Can Heal Your Life.* Hays House. Santa Monica, Ca.

Larson, B. (1981). *There's More to Health Than Not Being Sick.* Word Books. Waco, Texas.

Lesham, L. (1977) *You Can Fight for Your Life.* M. Evans & Co. New York, N.Y.

Padus, E. (1986) *Your Emotions and Your Health.* Rodal Press. Emmas, Pa.

Schindler, J. (1954). *How To Live 365 Days a Year.* Fawcett Crest Books. Greenwich, Cn.

(Other books referred to will appear in the bibliography at the conclusion of the book.)

Chapter Sixteen
Miscellaneous Information

(1) Durbin Inducted into International Hypnosis Hall of Fame (from a news release by Joanie Kingsley, 1992)

Reverend Paul G. Durbin of New Orleans, Louisiana, was presented with the Hypnotherapist "SEALAH" Award at the 13th. Annual "SEALAH" Awards Dinner held during the International Hypnosis Hall of Fame Annual Conference. The honor was presented to Durbin by Penny Duton Rafa, Founder of the IHHF and Robert "Bert" Freeman, Executive Vice President of IHHF. The Awards Dinner was one of the Highlights of the conference which was held at Guest Quarters Hotel, Plymouth Meeting, Pa.

Durbin is a United Methodist Minister serving as Director of Pastoral Care at Pendleton Memorial Methodist Hospital in New Orleans, La (Biography followed as of 1992) . . . He is consulted by medical doctors for pain management, stress management, and stop smoking for in-patients and out-patients. He also works with clients for those areas plus overcoming phobias, weight control and other means of self improvement.

The IHHF presents each year the prestigious "SEALAH" Awards. The "SEALAH" Awards are presented to individuals and/or organizations for outstanding contributions and achievements. Three other nominees were selected for "SEALAH" Awards among the 18 who were proposed for these honors. In addition to Durbin, inducted were: Helen Acord who received the "SEALAH" Pioneer Award, Wendell G. Loder who received the "SEALAH" Lifetime Achievement Award, and St. John's University, Springfield, La. received the "SEALAH" Education Award accepted by University President Dr. Arthur Winkler.

(2) Durbin Named NBHA "FELLOW" Inside Methodist 1993

Methodist Hospital Chaplain Paul G. Durbin Ph.D. has been named a Fellow of the National Board of Hypnotherapy of Hypnotic Anesthesiology (NBHA), the highest level of recognition conferred by the Board. He is one of nine in the country to receive this distinction.

"Recognition by NBHA is an honor which comes with hours of study, training, and years of experience," says Chaplain Durbin. "Hypnotherapy techniques are proving successful in treating an increasing number of medical conditions and I am pleased to utilize those techniques with appropriate patients." NBHA is one of the nation's most respected professional organizations due to the high standard required for membership. The organization recognizes competence demonstrated by professional experience and training, and by passing the NBHA examination in the areas of educational hypnosis and/or hypnotherapy.

Recognition as a Fellow is restricted to health care professionals who meet the extensive requirements to be named a Registered Hypnotic Anesthesiologist and hold at least a Bachelors Degree from recognized college or university. Fellow applicants must submit a thesis length paper on any aspect of hypnotherapy based on original research or clinical practice experience. Chaplain Durbin received the Fellow of the NBHA honor from Methodist Hospital, President Fred Young.

(3) Durbin Named NACH Diplomat

At the 1994 National Association of Clergy Hypnotherapy Convention held in Chicago, Ill., Chaplain Paul G. Durbin, Ph.D. was named Diplomat. Diplomat is the highest honor awarded by NACH and Durbin was only the fifth person so honored. Chaplain Durbin, Pendleton Memorial Methodist Hospital, Director of Pastoral Care, had been on the Board of Directors since 1986, was "Member of the Year" for 1986-87.

(4) Disappointment Becomes a Blessing

(From Sybil Waldrop's Book, Getting Good at Being You)

In the summer of 1969, Major Paul Guy Durbin, a Chaplain in the United States Army, was assigned to a unit at Fort Hood, Texas. For his year and a half as Administrative Chaplain, he received the Meritorious Service Medal. Then he was transferred to another brigade to serve as Assistant Chaplain. Someone who rated his services from personnel put a derogatory remark on his Officers Efficiency Report (OER). Six months later while in training at Walter Reed Army Hospital, Major Durbin learned about the derogatory remark in his OER. He sent a disclaimer and requested that the unjust statement be removed. He was informed that the statement would remain, but the disclaimer would be part of the report.

In 1975 while serving in Bangkok, Thailand, Durbin received word that he had been passed over for promotion to Lieutenant Colonel, the derogatory remark was the culprit. According to policy if he was passed over again in 1976, he would leave the army.

Durbin's clinical training at Walter Reed Hospital prepared him emotionally for what otherwise would have been a grave disappointment. Prior to his clinical training, Major Durbin confessed that he had an inferiority complex which he described as a feeling of "low self-worth masked over with an outgoing personality." He had what he called a conversion experience. His motivation for ministry changed from fear to love. He developed a feeling of self-worth and dignity within himself which was not dependent upon verification from others although, admittedly, that helped and still does.

Major Durbin shared his plight with the Bishop of the Louisiana Conference. In June of 1976, while attending annual conference, Major Durbin was asked if he were interested in an opening at Pendleton Memorial Methodist Hospital in New Orleans beginning September 1. His clinical training at Walter Reed had prepared him for the work of hospital chaplain. Then Major Durbin received word that the military had declared the two boards had been illegally convened, and all officers passed over in 1975 and 1976 could stay on active duty until January, at which time their records would be reviewed again. Now he had a choice. Durbin chose to accept the position at Pendleton Memorial Methodist Hospital. In December of 1976, the army promotion board promoted Major Durbin to Lieutenant Colonel. He was to return to duty with his promotion date retroactive to 1975. He chose to remain at Pendleton Memorial Methodist Hospital.

While continuing his work at Pendleton Memorial Methodist Hospital, Major Durbin also became a chaplain in the Louisiana National Guard and was promoted to Lieutenant Colonel, and after attending staff school, he was promoted to full Colonel in 1984.

In February 1986, Colonel Durbin was informed that he was being considered for a new position as Army National Guard Special Assistant to the Army Chief of Chaplains which carried the rank of Brigadier General. In June, Durbin was selected but he could not wear the rank until federal recognition by Congress. He is now the first Brigadier General Chaplain in history of the Army National Guard. In telling me his story, the Chaplain recalled the story of Joseph. Joseph's brothers sold him into slavery and told their father that Joseph had been killed. Years passed, and a famine prompted Joseph's brothers to travel to Egypt to get grain. Unknowing to the brothers, Joseph was in charge of Egypt's grain. The Chaplain found solace in these words, "But Joseph said to them, 'Do not be afraid, for I am in God's place. And as for you, you meant evil against me, but God meant it for good in order to bring about this present result, to preserve many people alive' (Gen. 50:19-20)."

(5) Managing Stress Advertisement

(from Wellspring Newsletter July, 1994)

Stress is the body's response to a demand placed upon it. It is the tension you feel when faced with a new, unpleasant, or threatening situation. Stress can produce an automatic reaction to a danger or a demand. Muscles tighten, blood pressure rises, and heart rate increases as the body prepares itself for "fight" or "flight." Stress is also essential to life and is often considered "The spice of life." Some degree of stress can be good since it inspires you to meet life's challenges. It is only when it becomes excessive that it can be harmful to both your physical and mental health. Instead of feeling nervous, angry, upset, or burned out, you feel calm, happy, in control, and alive by managing your stress.

Begin by doing something just for you. Do something you enjoy and set aside some time just for you. For example, take a hobby; do it with commitment—this means stick to it. You should be able to see and feel the difference.

Other things you may choose to include are physical exercise, deep breathing, self-hypnosis, and/or meditation. You may also need to get more sleep, work out anger, talk out problems, eat well, manage your time better, and take breaks. All of these suggestions imply you helping you.

- *STRESS MANAGEMENT:* 7:00 P.M.—8:30 P.M. Reverend Paul G. Durbin, Ph.D.
  Director of Pastoral Care Pendleton Memorial Methodist Hospital, will explore ways of reducing stress through imagery, self-hypnosis and relaxation techniques. Lecture, discussion, and demonstration will be included (Wednesday July 13)
- *SELF-HELP THROUGH SELF-HYPNOSIS:* 7:00 P.M.—8:30 P.M. This program is designed to explore the methods of self-hypnosis for self-improvement. It focuses on myths as well as the positive use of hypnosis and will include demonstration and participation. Presented by Reverend Paul G. Durbin (Wednesday July 20)

- *STOP SMOKING WITH HYPNOSIS:* (By individual appointment)
  Become a non-smoker through the use of relaxation, imagery, and hypnosis. Reverend Paul G. Durbin will conduct individual sessions. By fee. For more information and/or reservations, call the Chaplains office—244-5430. ("Wellspring" is the Pendleton Memorial Methodist Hospital logo for community education. Stress Management and Self Hypnosis class are offered to the public each July and January. These are among the best attended classes offered by Wellspring.)

(6) Smoke Free Facility Letter by Mr. Fred Young, Jr.

(President of Pendleton Memorial Methodist Hospital)

Dear Employee:

As you may be aware, Methodist Hospital will become a smoke-free facility on September 1st. The smoke-free environment includes Methodist Hospital, the Methodist Cancer Center, Methodist Ambulatory Surgery Center, Methodist Health System Foundation, Physical Medicine Center, and the Child Care Center.

The move to a smoke-free environment supports the position of the Hospital Medial Staff and the Orleans Parish Medical Society, calling for all health care facilities to eliminate opportunities for smoking. There will be two designated areas outside the facility where smoking will be allowed. The sun deck on the fourth floor near the Chapel and the gazebo in back of the hospital across from the emergency department will be designated as smoking areas. In addition, for the Methodist Cancer Center and Methodist Ambulatory Surgery Center, special areas outside these buildings will be noted.

Hospital Chaplain Paul Durbin will also conduct one-on-one hypnosis sessions to help smokers break the habit. Please contact the Chaplain's Office at extension 5430 for additional information.

As you know, smoking is a leading and proven contributing factor to heart disease, respiratory illness and lung cancer. Recent research indicates that those who do not smoke, but are in the company of heavy smokers, are just as susceptible.

As a leading health care facility and corporate citizen of New Orleans East, Methodist Hospital must set an example of a healthy environment so that others may follow. In the coming weeks, you will be learning more about the Hospital's campaign to eliminate smoking. For those of you who are smokers, I encourage you to participate in one or more of the smoking cessation programs that will be offered.

Sincerely,

Fred Young, President

(7) Letter to Physicians Concerning Hypnosis

TO: Methodist Hospital Medical Staff
FROM: Chaplain Paul G. Durbin, Ph.D.
SUBJECT: Stop Smoking, Stress Management, Pain Management, Weight Control, and other self-improvement procedures through the use of relaxation, positive imagery, and hypnosis.

A number of physicians on the staff of Pendleton Memorial Methodist Hospital have requested information concerning stop smoking, stress management, pain management, weight control and other self-improvement procedures. The client receives a booklet, *Introduction to the Value of Hypnosis,* and a tape on the subject which has been identified to help reinforce suggestions given during the session.

STOP SMOKING: The Stop Smoking Program has been very successful. The program usually takes one session with a free follow-up session within 30 days if needed. The hour consists of a discussion of what hypnosis is and is not, and how hypnosis helps one overcome the smoking habit. The client's smoking history is discussed and reason why client desires to be a non-smoker. After determining the client's response patterns, the hypnosis begins with proper suggestions for being a non-smoker.

STRESS MANAGEMENT: Stress Management for an individual may take one to several sessions. Discussion of stress factor, how to better deal with them, and progressive relaxation and self-hypnosis are taught to the client.

PAIN MANAGEMENT: I am available upon request to teach patients progressive relaxation, positive imagery and self-hypnosis for pain management. The procedures are used in conjunction with client's medical care and requires a doctor's referral.

WEIGHT CONTROL: In regards to the "Weight Control" Program, a doctor's referral is required. I do not provide a diet plan as I am not a dietitian or medical doctor. Three sessions for weight control counseling are required with more available if needed.

I am a Certified Clinical Hypnotherapist and a Diplomat with the National Association of Clergy Hypnotherapist, a Fellow with the

National Board of Hypnotherapy and Hypnotic Anesthesiology (NBHA) and the American Association of Professional Hypnotherapist (AAPH). I have written many articles for Professional Journals, given seminars throughout the United States on Hypnosis, and was inducted into the International Hypnosis Hall of Fame in 1992, located in Blue Bell, Pa. I received the *Pen and Quill* Award from NBHA for my book *Human Trinity Hypnotherapy,* in 1994.

Enclosed are copies of "Stop Smoking with Hypnosis" (Stress Management, Pain Management, and Weight Control) for your office.

(8) Stop Smoking with Hypnosis (Stress Management, Pain Management, Weight Control)

Chaplain Paul G. Durbin, Ph.D., Director of Pastoral Care, Pendleton Memorial Methodist Hospital, is a Certified Clinical Hypnotherapist who is available to help you overcome the smoking habit. Chaplain Durbin's "Stop Smoking with Hypnosis" Program usually takes one session with a free follow-up within 30 days if needed.

The hour consists of a discussion of what hypnosis is and is not and how hypnosis helps one overcome the smoking habit. The client's smoking history is discussed and reason why the client desires to be a non-smoker. After determining the client's response patterns, the hypnosis begins with proper suggestions for being a non-smoker. The client receives a booklet, "Introduction to the Value of Hypnosis" and a "Stop Smoking" audio tape to help reinforce suggestions given during the session.

For outpatient sessions, a donation to the Methodist Hospital Chaplain's Fund is recommended using a sliding scale based upon income. Senior Focus Members and Senior Citizens are recommended to donate at the lowest figure of the sliding scale. Donations are tax-deductible.

Chaplain Durbin is also available for Stress Management, Pain Management, Weight Control, Positive Imagery, and other improvement procedures. Pain Management and Weight Control requires a physician's referral.

Chaplain Durbin has written many articles for Professional Journals, presented seminars throughout the United States on Hypnosis, and was inducted in the International Hypnosis Hall of Fame in 1992, located in Blue Bell, Pa.

For questions and referrals, call Methodist Hospital Chaplain's Office at 244-5430.

(9) Hypnotist Teaches Students to Relax

(Nunez Community College Article)

By: Julie Landry, New Orleans Times-Picayune 1992

If the students in Paul Durbin's class at Nunez Community College in Chalmette look like they're sleeping, it's because he's doing a good job.

Durbin is Chaplain and Director of Pastoral Care at Pendlcton Memorial Methodist Hospital in New Orleans. He started using hypnosis to treat patients with chronic pain in 1981.

In a recent class, Durbin's students paired up to wind each other down in a progressive relaxation exercise. The hypnotist wooed the student into a dreamlike state by asking him to visualize a lemon. Richard Gardache, 45, of Chalmette waved his hands dramatically as he lulled Christine Pattini, 37, of Slidell to a quiet state.

"Can you see the lemon? Can you see it?" "Yes." "You're visionary. That's good," he said as Prattini closed her eyes. "I want you to take three deep breaths. You're going to relax. You're going to feel peace," he said.

Prattini's legs, crossed at the ankles, relaxed slightly. The fingers on her outstretched hand rested lightly on her legs, "All your tensions are going away. Now just enjoy the sensations," he said before slowly counting her back to an alert state. "Despite the distractions," Prattini said, indicating the 20 students surrounding her in the classroom, "I did feel relaxed."

Gardacher, who served 2 years as a New Orleans Police officer, uses the relaxation techniques to relieve chronic back pain but said he could've used these skills on the job. "Sometimes we used relaxation techniques with prisoners when they got out of hand." he said.

Ginger Frolich, 43, of Chalmette suffers from chronic pain in her legs and back. She has gotten relief from being hypnotized and wants to learn the technique herself. "I usually can sleep only an hour and a half at a time," she said. "This technique refreshes you and relaxes your whole body. It's like a booster shot."

"Often patients don't like to think they've been hypnotized," Durbin said. "They say they feel better and are more relaxed."

In one class exercise, Durbin swung a pendulum to show students how the direction that it swung could indicate answers to questions posed to someone under hypnosis. "It's not going to tell the future and not going to give you numbers on the lottery ticket but it will help you answer questions in your subconscious mind." he said.

Durbin said some people are afraid of hypnosis because they're worried the hypnotist will make them do something against their will. "The person (under hypnosis) is in control," Durbin said. "They won't do anything against their belief system to go under," Durbin said, "The person has to be able to think, reason, and communicate. You actually gain control, because hypnosis lets you learn more ways to improve your life."

(10) Four Brain Wave Patterns

There are four primary brain wave patterns: Beta, Alpha, Theta, and Delta. The *Beta* state is one of awakened physical alertness. This is the state in which we spend most of our waking time. The *Alpha* state brings heightened creativity and enhanced physical relaxation. The Alpha state produces hypnosis or deep meditation. *Theta* state is being on the brink of going to sleep. It is also a natural state of hypnosis. The *Delta* state is a state of light to profound sleep.

(11) Visual, Auditory, Kinesthetic

1. *Visual:* They usually speak in terms of seeing or watching. Examples: I see what you mean. I can't see that. Looks good. Picture this. Visual people will give vivid descriptions of things as though painting a picture. They have a tendency to show you something as they're talking. They like to have eye contact. Typically, a visual person will use predicates such as: see, behold, observe, view, witness, look, glance, etc. When a visual person thinks, his eyes tend to move up and to the right.
2. *Auditory:* You can recognize an auditory person by observing the way his eyes stay level while moving right and left, down and to the left. Auditories use "sound" words to communicate and they like the sound of their own voice. Their voices have an even, rhythmic, tempo and melodious, easy-to-listen-to-sound. They use terms like I hear what you say. That sounds good to me. They make lots of noise jingle coins or keys in the pocket, scuffle feet, walk loudly. They like to repeat things. If you ask them "What time is it?" they may repeat the question and then give you the answer. They laugh at the punch line and then repeat it. They don't need the eye to eye contact that visual people need. Typically an auditory person speaks using predicates such as listen, hear, take in, hark, attend, etc.

3. *Kinesthetic:* Kinesthetics' eyes move down and right when they are processing information. They readily express feelings about anything. They like or hate; they're hot or cold. You will hear "spaces" in kinesthetic's conversation while she/he takes time to check out his feelings about what is going on. The kinesthetic's voice is generally deeper than the voice of the visual or Auditories.

   Kinesthetic people will talk in terms of feelings. Examples: I can't handle this. I can't grasp that. I feel like a steak today. That doesn't feel right. They have a tendency to touch a lot, and they have a need to be touched back. Typically, a kinesthetic person will use predicates such as touch, handle, feel, itch, excite, sharpen, etc.

Most people have a dominate preference but can communicate in more than one mode. Knowing a person's mode helps you to communicate more effectively with him and to gain trust and rapport quickly. To be most effective, alter your response mode to that of the client. The knowledge of the client's mode help in formulating suggestions for the client.

(12) The Dark Mile: Coming Through a Bad Experience

Dr. Richard H. Hutton told of an interesting incident that he and a companion had during a visit to Scotland. They did most of their traveling by foot. Late one afternoon, they came to a little inn where they spent the night. As they were talking to the innkeeper, he told them that the most beautiful lake in all of Scotland was only about four miles from the inn. He got a map and traced the path to the lake with his finger. The path went around in a semi-circle. Dr. Hutton asked, "Isn't there a shorter way?" The innkeeper answered, "There is a shorter way, but no one goes that way by choice. It runs through the 'dark mile' which is a fearful gorge." Dr. Hutton desired to know why it was called the "dark mile." He was told that the path through the gorge was narrow and gloomy, dark and frightening, and that big overhanging ledges of rock was dripping water all along the way.

Wanting to save time, Dr. Hutton and his friend decided to go to the lake by way of the "dark mile." They found it about as the innkeeper had described it. Though they were both fearful, they were able to keep going because they gave each other support. They slowly made their way through the dark gorge and finally they saw the light that marked the end of the "dark mile." It had been gloomy, dark and frightening, but they had made it. As they came out of the gorge, before them was beautiful Lake Lackrey. Both gasped at the sight of the beautiful lake which was surrounded by the mountains. Dr. Hutton's friend said, "I don't believe that we would ever have appreciated the beauty of the lake if we hadn't traveled the 'dark mile'."

Each of us must at one time or another travel the "dark mile." You may feel that you are traveling that "dark mile" right now because of this problem. Use whatever faith you have to make it through your "dark mile" to the beauty of a new direction in your life.

(13) Buddha and the Man Who Wanted Deliverance

From 1973-75, I lived in the Buddhist nation of Thailand and there is an interesting story connected with Gautoma Buddha which I would like to share with you. Gautoma Buddha vowed that he would die unless he could find the way of life, the path of deliverance. The story is told that after he had found what he considered the way of life, a certain man came asking Buddha to show him the way. Buddha led the man down to the river. The seeker assumed that he was to undergo some act of purification or baptism. When they were some distance out in the stream, Buddha suddenly grabbed the man and pushed his head under the water. In a last minute effort, the man pulled himself free and quickly brought his head out of the water. Buddha asked him, "When you thought you were going to drown, what did you want most?" The man gasped, "Air." Back came Buddha, "When you want deliverance as badly as you wanted air, then you will get it." It seems that what we truly want and work for, we tend to get.

(14) Sir Henry Vane of London and Priorities

As we look at our world today, we see that many have failed to get their priorities in order. Many are like Sir Henry Vane of London. Sir Henry was to have his head cut off at the executioner's block. He was given one last word. Rather than pleading for his life or making some great statements, he begged the executioner not to hit a painful boil on his neck. How ridiculous we might say for once that ax feel it did not matter what part of the neck it hit. He magnified the insignificant and overlooked the vital. How often do we magnify the insignificant and overlook the vital.

(15) Airplane Metaphor for Experiencing New Situations

When we are faced with a course of action that seems unfamiliar to us, we often think that because we have not experienced the exact situation before, we know nothing about it. In those circumstances, it may be useful to think of the situation in the same way as someone might who is about to take a trip on an airplane for the first time. He or she may think that they know nothing about it, but they may discover that they know quiet a bit about it. Let's say that this person is Mr. Jones.

Mr. Jones may never have been on an airplane before, but has been on a bus. Furthermore, he has been on a bus going to different town so he knows how to read a timetable and find out about departure and arrival times. Having done that, he knows how to get in touch with the travel agency for buying tickets. He knows how to phone ahead to make sure that the plane is going to leave on time.

In the past, when he was traveling by bus, he knew how to find the right place to board the bus. He had some suitcases, so he knew how to get them to the place where they will be check for the journey. In the bus, he chatted in a comfortable, friendly way with the people sitting next to him. At the end of the journey, he know how to find the special place to pick up the suitcases and to make his way through the bus depot where the taxis are or to meet this friends to pick him up.

Mr. Jones had never been on an airplane, but he had traveled before on commercial transportation so he could use the knowledge to help him on this trip. In fact, Mr. Jones knows almost all there is to know about traveling on an airplane except actually being on an airplane. It is just all of this information was scattered around in a variety of different experiences, and needed to be gathered up and re-applied to the new circumstances.

For this present situation in which you find yourself, ask your subconscious mind to gather up all the information it can find that may in someway relate to it . . . A little bit of information from that past experience, more information from another experience . . . And put them all together in one package . . . One that is useful and appropriate for the present. You know far more than you know that you know. Enjoy discovering the wonderful range of your own knowledge.

(16) Overcoming Procrastination with "Sleeping Well on a Windy Night"

You have made a decision to overcome procrastinating because you want to be on time and succeed in life. You expect to do things on time and you feel a sense of enthusiasm and confidence in living your new attitude toward getting things done.

You are overcoming procrastinating because you want to . . . You are taking a great deal of pride in the fact that you have matured . . . You are taking control of your life and beginning to do the things that you put off in the past . . . You exchange your old habit of putting it off to your new approach of getting it done. You are ready to do the unpleasant task which you used to put off doing and you feel good about yourself. You refuse to let tasks pile up on you anymore. You get it done.

You complete your task easily and you have confidence in yourself and abilities. You get the job done well, efficiently, and properly. You stop worrying about the job you need to do and get it done. You are pleased with yourself for doing what needs to be done. You enjoy a feeling of success in each and every task that you take on and finish. As your confidence grows, as your abilities grow, as you accomplish, more and more every day, you feel good about yourself and your self-confidence increases more and more everyday and in every way.

I share with you this story: A boy went to a farmer and asked to be given a job working on the farm. The farmer asked, "Are you willing to work?" "Yes sir, I can sleep well on a windy night," was his strange reply. "Can I trust you to look after my things?" Again the boy replied, "Yes sir, I can sleep well on a windy night." The farmer asked several questions seeking to determine if the boy was honest and trustworthy, but to each question, he got the one reply.

He decided the boy might be a little foolish, but there was something about him that the farmer liked, so he hired him. The boy proved to be a good worker and everything went well until one night a big storm came up. The farmer rushed to the boy's room. "Get up," he shouted, "Let's go tie down the hay stacks, put up the tools and secure the barn door." But the boy was so sound asleep that the farmer could not wake him. Fearing to waste time trying to get him up, he rushed out to see about the things.

When he came to the hay stacks, he found them already firmly tied. He found the tools in their proper places in the barn and doors closed securely. As he went back into the house he realized what the boy had meant about sleeping well on a windy night. He meant that each day, he did as best he could and, even in the midst of the storm, he could sleep.

By coming to me, you have made a commitment to overcome procrastination. You get things done so you can "sleep well on a windy night."

(17) Durbin Elected President of NACH

Chaplain Paul Durbin, director of pastoral care at Pendleton Memorial Methodist Hospital, has been elected president of the National Association of Clergy Hypnotherapists.

The association provides support for clergy who want to increase their skill in the pastoral use of hypnosis. Durbin has been on the group's board of directors since 1986 and was named its member of the year for 1986-87.

Chapter Seventeen
Suggestibility, Imagery, and Healing Stories

(1) Suggestibility

The mind, conscious and subconscious, is greatly influenced by suggestion. Suggestibility is a natural characteristic of our humanity. It is the foundation of learning and change in our life. It is used in education, worship, politics, advertisement and human relations.

Stop for a moment to consider the power of words as one method of conveying suggestions. By words, the preacher proclaims the Good News of Faith. By words, thoughts are imparted from one person to another or from one generation to another. There are words that make us laugh and words that make us cry, words that bless and words that curse, words that honor and words that condemn, words that wound and words that heal. The old saying, "Sticks and stones may break my bones but words will never hurt me," is a false statement. Words can be helpful or harmful depending upon the way they are given and received.

Mr. Claud had heart by-pass surgery at another hospital, but he was admitted at Methodist Hospital about a month later. Thought the surgery had been successful, Mr. Claud's condition was progressively deteriorating. I was consulted by his physician to work with in regards to his attitude and lack of hope. During a hypnotic session, I asked him to go back to the beginning of his problem. He went back to his surgery. (A note about heart by-pass surgery; after the by-pass is completed, another surgeon normally closes the procedure with stitches.) As the by-pass doctor had completed his procedure, he said, "I have done all I can do—sew him up." He meant that he had completed his portion and the other surgeon could now close up the wound. Though under anesthesia, Mr. Claud heard him and thought the doctor meant, "It was so bad, I can't help him, sew him up." I explained the procedure and asked him to look at it from a different understanding. Now, he could begin the process of healing. That occurred about five years ago and Mr. Claud is active and healthy.

My mother was in a hospital in Shreveport, La. for the removal of a cancerous growth on her jaw. She had surgery and had returned to her room. I stayed with her from about three in the afternoon until about ten the next morning. The nurses were very responsive to my mother's calls for the longest that she had to wait for a nurse to come was about three minutes. I consider that excellent response time. The first thing that each nurse and her doctor said when they came into the room for whatever reason was, "Mrs. Durbin are you hurting?" Until about nine that night my mother had not needed anything for pain and I wondered, "Would she needed any pain medication at nine, had the question been different." What if the nurses and doctor had said something like, "Mrs. Durbin, are you comfortable?" "Mrs. Durbin, how are you feeling?" Instead the suggestion that they were reinforcing with each visit was that my mother should be experiencing pain.

During that same hospital stay, the IV needed changing from one hand to the other. The nurse who came to make the change said, "Mrs. Durbin I wish I had an anesthetic to give you so that this would not be so painful." I said, "Oh you can give her an anesthetic." She responded, "No, no, I would get in trouble for I do not have a doctor's order for an anesthetic." I replied, "Just watch and see." I took my mother's hand and said, "Look at me mother while the nurse works on your other hand. In a moment, the nurse will apply an *antiseptic* swab to your other hand. You feel the cold *antiseptic* as it is applied. The cold *antiseptic* causes a numbing effect so that you feel only pressure." As I talked to my mother the nurse completed her mission of inserting the IV. When I stopped talking, my mother turned her head toward the nurse and said, "When are you going to begin?" The nurse looked surprised and said, "Mrs. Durbin, I have already put the IV in your hand and I am now putting the tape on to hold it in place." I said, "I told you that you could administer an anesthetic without a doctor's prescription." In both these illustrations concerning my mother's nurses, you can see the power of suggestion. No formal hypnotic induction was used, but in both cases hypnotic effect was accomplished: one negative and one positive.

Whatever use is made of hypnosis, whether it is in therapy, clinical research, relief of symptoms, or merely for amusement, we cannot get away from the fact that none of it would be possible without the use of suggestion. Suggestion is used to induce the hypnotic state; suggestion is used to control the responses while the person is hypnotized, suggestion is used to attain responses after the session has been completed, and suggestion is used to get the person out of the hypnotic state. In other words, the entire procedure of hypnosis, from pre-induction to attainment of the individual's purpose for using hypnosis, is all founded on suggestion. Therefore the proper use of suggestion is the most important aspects of hypnosis. The word "suggestion" used in hypnotic context, is the acceptance of an idea or belief to the point of causing changes in an individual's actions, body responses, attitudes, emotions, or characteristics.

Some people respond better to direct suggestions, while others respond best to indirect suggestion. Most of us can respond to both direct and indirect suggestion but generally have a preference for one or the other. Because I believe in the importance of an individual's suggestibility, I have everyone who comes to my office for counseling fill out a suggestibility questionnaire which will generally give an indication of their dominate response. When working with a hospital patient instead of using the suggestibility cessionaire, I ask questions to help me determine the dominate form of suggestibility for the patient.

Our suggestibility usually comes from our primary care giver (usually our mother). If the child experiences his/her mother as saying what she means and meaning what she says, he/she will usually be more responsive to direct suggestions. If the verbal and non-verbal parts of her communication does not express the same thing, the child begins to search for the real meaning. He/she begins to look for the implied meaning rather than what is actually said. Balanced suggestibility comes when in certain areas, the mother is consistent in what she said while in other areas, she gave conflicting messages.

I tend to be close to the middle with a slight dominance for direct suggestion for when my mother told me not to do something, I knew she meant it. If she told me to do something, then I should do it. There was a cause and effect. Mother laid down the law and I followed it or I reaped the consequences. On the other hand, mother could be indirect in her request. She might say to me, "Paul don't you think you should go visit Mrs. Smith. She is sick and she gave you a gift for Christmas last year." Now that sounds like I had a choice but I did not. She meant for me to go se Mrs. Smith and if my answer to her was "no," she would let me know in no uncertain terms that I was to go.

(2) Semantics: The Meaning of Words

When we give suggestions to clients, we assume that we are being understood. Words have different meanings. We need to be sure that the client is understanding the meaning we are trying to present. Remember that the subconscious mind tends to take statements literally. A hypnotherapist who had worked with many people for weight control used a statement, "You are reducing down to 120 lbs." The woman was reducing but her hips were getting bigger. Her subconscious took reducing down to mean that the fat was going to her hips. After he realized what was happening, he changed his words and she reached her desired weight of 120 lbs. with a nice figure. She was the only one out of many who this man worked with who responded as such, but it shows how people may accept a meaning different that what we mean.

I am going to say a word and you think of a meaning. I will then use the word in a sentence and see if your meaning and my meaning are the same.

1. **BUG**—The judge gave the police permission to bug the suspect's phone.
2. **COOL**—He remained cool in the midst of the heated argument.
3. **HIGH**—He was arrested for being high on cocaine.
4. **POT**—If you would like to eat, there is a pot of peas on the stove.
5. **DOG**—After working all day, I was dog tired.
6. **MAKE OUT**—She had to make out four different applications.
7. **FIRE**—He had to fire Bill because he hit a customer.
8. **BOOK**—The cop said, "I am going to book you for robbery."
9. **SPEED**—His head is all messed up because of using speed.
10. **SCREW**—He has a screw loose.
11. **HIP**—He is really hip.

I believe that you can see by this exercise that we depend on the context of our sentences and non-verbal cues to give meaning to our words. Our non-verbal communication usually serves to intensify word's meaning. Remember, words and imagery are the most important tool in the field of hypnotherapy.

We act and feel not necessarily according to what things are really like, but according to the image our mind holds of what they are like. We have certain mental images of ourself, our world, the people around us, of God, and we behave as though these images were the truth whether they are or not.

As an illustration, if a husband asks his wife the question, "Where is my blue and white tie?" The wife may respond according to how she hears the question. If she hears it as a little boy saying, "Mama, where is my tie?" She may respond, "You must learn to keep up with your things." If she hears him speak as a domineering parent, she might respond, "Why are you always picking on me? It is not my responsibility." If she hears his question as a simple request for information, she may respond, "I believe you put it on the hanger with your blue suit."

Her reaction did not necessarily come from the requested information, but how she heard the question.

When formulating suggestions, remember the nature of communication. Words create mental images in the mind of the person to whom we are speaking. The success of getting the person to understand the meaning we intend is dependent on whether we are creating the same mental image in the person's mind who hears our words. A good hypnotist attempts to consider each client on an individual basis and attempts to recognize the different reaction and adapt to them. With this in mind, I share with you the following story concerning communication.

(3) Communication: The Buddhist Temple

The monks of a Buddhist Temple in Japan would allow anyone to spend the night who could win an argument about Buddhism with one of the monks that lived there. If the traveler is defeated in the argument, he has to move on. In the Buddhist Temple, two brother monks were dwelling together. The older one was learned, but the younger one was stupid and had only one eye.

A wandering monk came and asked for lodging, properly challenging the monks to a debate about the sublime teaching. The elder brother, tired that day from much studying, told the younger one to take his place. He said to both that they were to carry the dialogue in silence. So the young monk and the stranger went to the shrine and sat down.

Shortly afterward the traveler rose and went in to the elder brother and said: "Your young brother is a wonderful fellow, he defeated me." "Relate the dialogue to me." "Well," explained the traveler, "First I held up one finger, representing Buddha, the enlightened one. So he held up two fingers signifying Buddha and his teaching. I held up three fingers, representing Buddha, his teaching, and his followers, living a harmonious life. Then he shook his clenched first in my face, indicating that all three come from one realization. Thus, he won and so I have no right to remain here." With this, the traveler left.

"Where is that fellow?" asked the younger one, running in to his older brother who said, "I understand you won the debate." "Won nothing, I'm going to beat him up." "Tell me the subject of the debate," asked the elder one. "Why the minute he saw me he held up one finger, insulting me by reminding me that I have only one eye. Since he was a stranger I thought I would be polite to him, so I held up two fingers congratulating him for having two eyes. Then the impolite man held up three fingers suggesting that between us we only have three eyes. So, I got mad and started to punch him, but he ran out and ended it."

(I heard this story in a seminar by Reverend Randy VanNostrand at the National Association of Clergy Hypnotherapists some years ago.) A paraphrase of that story maybe, "I know that you believe you understood what you think I said, but I am not sure you realize that what you heard is not what I meant."

(4) Imagery and Healing Stories

Imagery is a flow of thoughts you may see, hear, feel, smell, or taste. An image is an inner representation of your experience, of your fantasies—a way your mind codes, stores, and expresses information. Imagery is made up of the dreams and daydreams; memories and reminiscence; plans, projections, and possibilities. It is the language of the emotions and most important of the deeper self.

Imagery is a window on your inner world; a way of viewing your own ideas, feelings, and interpretations. Imagination, in this sense, is not sufficiently valued in our culture for imaginary is often equated with the fanciful, the unreal, and the impractical. In school, we are taught the three R's while creativity, uniqueness, and interpersonal skills are either barely tolerated or frankly discouraged. As adults, we are usually paid to perform tasks and to think creatively. The premium is on the practical, the useful, the real as it should be-but imagination nurtures human reality as a water brings life to a desert.

Without imagination, civilization as we know it would not exist. It took imagination—the ability to conceive of new possibilities—to make fire, create weapons, and cultivate crops; to construct buildings, invent cars, airplanes, space shuttles, television, and computers.

The changes and learning that can take place through the use of imagery and healing stories are two of the most interesting aspects of communication with the subconscious.

Imagination and imagery helps the person's subconscious to understand there can be a better way. The possibility of change begins with the imagination. Inventions, music, writings, changes in behavior begins with imagination.

Imagery comes in two ways: visual and imagery. A visual person can see in the mind's eye as if viewing a scene in reality or on the TV screen of their mind. The visual person can also use their imagination. The non-visual person can not see pictures but they can imagine scenes, sound, and experience feelings.

Healing stories are used as an indirect suggestion for the client to hear and receive the meaning it has for him. Jesus used healing stories which we call parables to teach his message. The healing story allows the client to interpret the story and take responsibility for change.

The more one uses positive images in his mind, the easier it becomes for these images to become a reality. When images of health, success, and life styles changes are accepted by the subconscious mind, there is a tendency for the images to be realized. If you visualize or image yourself doing whatever it is you desire, you begin to act, do, think in ways to bring it about.

In 1985, I decided that I wanted to write a book on hypnosis and have it published. I wrote the book and began the process of finding a publisher. Each day, I would visualize my book and signing the book for someone who purchased it. It was accepted twice, but for various reasons, it had gone unpublished. During this time it was turned down by 30 publishers. I never gave up. I continued my visualization. Finally it was accepted and published by Access Publishing Company and was released in January 1994. That book was *Human Trinity Hypnotherapy.* After that I imaged this book being published and it is so.

In early 1986, I was informed that I was among five Army National Guard Chaplains throughout the nation being considered for promotion to Brigadier General. This was a new position so whoever was selected would be the first Army National Guard Chaplain to be promoted to Brigadier General. Each day, I visualized myself in my Generals uniform. I pictured the Chief of Chaplains of the Army pinning my star on my uniform. In May 1986, I was selected and became the first Army National Guard Chaplain to be promoted to general rank in the history of the nation.

I use imagery for many things and it has either worked or I am still in the process if imagining it into being. I still am working on being selected as a winner in the National Publisher's Sweepstakes, for I am still imagining that phone call or knock on the door with their representative informing me that I am a winner. Albert Einstein once said, "Imagination is the preview of coming events."

It could be said that the mother of your reality is your imagination. Norman Cousins said, "We move toward our expectations." Our expectations, thoughts, and imagination can and does affect our reality. There is a story of the great Renaissance artist Michelangelo, a famous statue, and a boy named, Giovanni. Every day after school, Giovanni would rush to Michelangelo's studio to watch the famous sculptor chip away at a 14-foot-high block of marble. Week after week, the boy came and watched, as the magnificent status of David was being formed. In all innocence, Giovanni ask Michelangelo, "How did you know he was in there?" Michelangelo knew because he had a vision of what he could create. If he was willing to dedicate himself to it if he was willing to work hard and long, enough, his vision would become a reality.

Maurice Maeterlinck tells of an interesting experience that thought him to envision the best for his life each day. While walking through the country one day, he stopped to admire a beautiful garden surrounded by a white fence. As he stood there a little old lady, showing her age, stopped by his side. After he greeted her, she came closer and asked if he was enjoying the flowers? When he said that he was, she launched upon a detailed description of the harmony of colors and shapes of each and every type of flower in the garden. When she concluded her vivid description, she looked up at him and he noticed that she was blind. He asked her how she was able to describe the vast array of colors to such perfection, inasmuch as she could not see. The old woman answered that when she was able to see, she learned to look at the beauties of nature as if she would never see them again. Her ancient vision was able to carry her through life. Though she could not see with her eyes, she could see with her mind.

(5) Explore Your Imagery Abilities (adapted from a Martin Rossman Script)

Begin by getting comfortable as you can . . . Let your eyes close and take three slow, deep breaths: breathing in relaxation and exhaling tension . . . Now take another deep, letting go kind of breath . . . Just begin to let go of any unnecessary tension, stress, anxiety, or discomfort . . . Begin to focus inside and let go . . . Let the images come as they will. It may be visual or just a feeling but let it happen.

As I ask you to imagine a variety of things, allow yourself to observe what happens for you . . . Remember, there is no right or wrong way to imagine these things . . . Just notice what it's like for you . . . That's your only responsibility now . . . Notice what it's like . . .

Visualize or imagine a sandy beach . . . Feel the warm breeze . . . Hear the sounds of the waves going in and going out . . . Walk along the beach . . . Imagine or see the beautiful blue sky with a few white clouds lazily drifting by . . . Hear the sounds of the waves going in and going out . . . Walk along the beach. Feel the sand between your toes as you walk along the beach . . . Imagine or see the beautiful blue sky with a few white clouds lazily drifting by . . . Hear the sound of birds as they fly over your head . . . Lie down on a blanket . . . Feel the warmth of the sun on your body and the warmth of the sand beneath the blanket . . .

Now let the image go . . . And let a square form in your mind's eye or on your mental screen . . . Any kind of square is fine . . . Just notice what it's like as you continue to observe it . . . Now let that image fade and imagine a circle . . . Notice how big or small it is, and how round . . . Let the circle be yellow . . . A bright yellow circle . . . Notice if it helps to think of the sun or a yellow lemon . . . Let the yellow fade and imagine the circle is red . . . Like an apple or something red that's familiar to you . . . Now let that go and imagine the circle is blue . . . Like the sky or the ocean . . . now let that image go . . . Imagine you are in the country, and it's wintertime . . . You are walking through the freshly fallen snow and can hear and feel it crunch beneath your boots . . . The air is cold and crisp, and you can see your breath as you exhale . . . In the distance a radio is playing . . . You go into a house and there is a fire place with wood logs burning bringing warmth to the room. You go over to the fireplace and warm your hands and feet . . . Feel the warmth, enjoy the warmth . . . Smell the coffee brewing and enjoy a hot cup of coffee . . .

Now let that image go . . . Imagine a very happy time in your childhood . . . Maybe you are at a party, playing with a friend, or just having a good time . . . Notice the sounds you hear, the things you see, and how you feel . . . Now let that go . . . and recall some time you felt very much at peace with yourself . . . A time when you felt very peaceful, very centered, and calm . . . Imagine it as if it were happening right now . . . Notice where you are . . . And your face . . . Your voice, especially notice the feeling of peacefulness and calm . . . Notice where you feel these qualities, and let them be there . . . Let them begin to grow in you . . . Let them amplify and expand, filling your whole body with feelings of peacefulness and calm . . . Let the feelings overflow your body to fill the space around you . . . so that all of you is bathed in the peacefulness . . .

Now slowly let yourself begin to become aware of the room . . . and let yourself come awake and alert, bringing back with you and feelings of peacefulness you may have experienced . . . Remember what was of interest or importance to you, and take some time to talk about it . . .

Evaluate your imagery experience.

Did you experience any of the images as pictures? Sounds? Smells? Tastes? Feelings? Which images came easily? Which were more difficult, and were there any you weren't able to imagine at all? Were you surprised by any particular images or your reactions to them?

Did you experience heat, cold, peace, or other sensations at any time? If you did, you've already begun to influence your body through your imagery. If not, you may want to experiment with your own images until you can imagine these sensations.

Chapter Eighteen
Guidelines, Rules of the Mind, Etc.

(1) Rules of the Mind

1. Every thought or idea causes a physical reaction.
2. What is expected tends to be realized (good or bad) "Whatsoever a person thinketh in their heart so is she/he." Worry is a form of negative programming. Job said "That which I feared has come upon me." The subconscious can not tell the difference between a wish and a fear.
3. Imagination is more powerful than knowledge. When dealing with the subconscious mind, reason is often overruled by imagination. Imagination is more powerful than will power.
4. Opposing ideas cannot be held at the same time. One or the other will become dominant.
5. Once an idea has been accepted by the subconscious mind that idea remains fixed until it is replaced with another idea.
6. Each suggestion acted upon creates a greater possibility for accepting successive suggestion.
7. A message to the subconscious connected to an emotional experiences has more power.
8. Law of Reverse Effect: (a) The harder you try to do something, the more difficult it is to do. (b) The greater the conscious effort, the less the subconscious response.

(2) Guidelines for Using Hypnosis

1. Develop rapport with the client before beginning hypnosis. Rapport is a bond of trust established between the hypnotist and the client. Trust fosters a willingness on the part of the client to cooperate and establishes a feeling of empathy on the part of thy hypnotist. Rapport is established by being sensitive to and concerned about the client's needs.
2. Even as a beginner, always exhibit confidence in what you are doing.

3. During the first session you have with a person, be sure to go over the nature and characteristics of hypnosis. Discuss misconceptions and answer any question the person may ask.

4. Regardless of what may come up after you have gone into a hypnotic induction with a client, always remain calm and continue talking in the same smooth tone of voice. Keep yourself under control at all times, even if the client begins crying or becomes hysterical. If you become excited or your tone of voice changes, you might lose contact with the client, by changing to a calm tone, the client can then adapt to your smooth, calm voice.

5. Never attempt to remove pain unless you know the cause of the pain and know for sure it can be removed without causing further injury to the client. Remember that pain is always there to let a person know something is wrong. For example, if a client has a stomach ache and you remove the pain, it could be his/her appendix and by eliminating the pain, the results could be tragic.

6. If you have a client who is experiencing difficulty into going into a hypnotic state, remain confident. Keep in mind that everyone can be hypnotized. Review what you have done. Perhaps you didn't clear up some misconception in the client's mind, or perhaps you made some statement the client's mind did not want to accept, or you may be using the wrong induction for that person.

7. If you are unsuccessful using hypnosis with an individual; never tell the person that he/she cannot be hypnotized. You may tell them that though you were unable to lead them into the hypnotic state on this occasion, they can be hypnotized because everyone who can think, reason, and communicate cab be hypnotized.

8. Never date or have a sexual affair with a person you are having hypnotic sessions with. It could ruin you reputation and is unethical. Remember that most people do not understand hypnosis and would believe you seduced the person through suggestions you had given while the person was hypnotized.

9. At all times when guiding a person into a hypnotic state, be calm and confident.

10. If someone is enjoying the hypnotic state so much that they are not ready to come out at this time, you may use one or more of several techniques. If time permits, you may say,"You can drift into a normal, natural sleep, awakening when it is appropriate or when someone wakes you up." You may say, "Your bladder is getting fuller and fuller. You need to go to the bathroom. Your bladder is getting fuller and fuller." If you are charging for a session, you may say, "You may remain in hypnosis as long as you desire, but in one minute from now, I will begin to charge one hour's cost for each minute you remain in hypnosis."

11. Develop the skill to be able to detect the cause of the difficulty and know how to handle it so you can aid the client in being released from the control it is having on her.

12. You must have a knowledge of enough hypnotic techniques that you can be flexible in your approach, so you will be able to use the best technique for the specific problem involved. Always proceed with an air of complete confidence. Give the impression of being an authority in hypnosis even if you are a beginner. Imagine how you might feel if you went to a surgeon to discuss a surgical procedure he was going to perform on you, and he said, "I'm glad you are ready for surgery. You will be my first patient, I hope this operation will be a success."

13. You must be able to handle your own shortcomings and biases without projecting them on to the client.

14. When a situation calls for an attempt to remove a symptom by suggestion, there is a way you can be sure to do so without causing any danger, and that is, when using the finger response technique by asking the question: "Is it okay for you to get rid of that symptom?" If the answer given by the subconscious mind is "yes" there will be no danger. If the answer is "no," you should not attempt to remove the symptom at that time.

    There have been critics who have said that if a symptom is removed, another symptom may appear but this is seldom true. If an aspirin is used to relieve a headache, does other symptoms develop? This illustration is used an example to let you know that symptom removed by hypnotic suggestion is no more dangerous than symptoms removed by any other treatment that does not eliminate the course of the problem. With hypnosis, the problem is often eliminated with the symptom.

15. As much as possible the surrounding should be concussive to relaxation and comfort. Pleasant lighting should be used if available, outside noises should be eliminated as much as possible. If disturbing noises should occur, just say, "Now allow the outside noises and sounds contribute to your experience of relaxation."

16. Close friends and relatives sitting in to observe may but not always interfere with the client's ability to concentrate. The client may wonder what they think about everything that is occurring. He may be wondering if they are going to think he looks silly, or if they will kid him after it's all over.

17. Never try to work in areas beyond your training and experience. Keep in mind, that some people who seek the aid of a hypnotist are neurotic, so you must always be prepared for the unexpected, and always observe rules of caution. Do not try to do therapy you are not qualified to handle.

18. Think of hypnosis as a science and work accordingly. By observing these rules, you will be able to succeed where many other hypnotists have failed.

19. Be sure that the client is brought out of the hypnotic state before she/he leaves your office. Always count out even if the client has their eyes open and may be talking to you.

20. Continue to read, study, go to seminars and courses on hypnosis so that you can continue to improve your knowledge and techniques.

(3) The Clinical Interview or Pre-Talk

The initial session with pre-induction interview or pre-talk is perhaps the most critical part of the hypnotic session. I have developed a very specific format which I have used successfully with thousands of clients. The purpose of the pre-talk is five fold:

1. To establish the purpose of the visit and determine the therapeutic objectives and to get to know the client and to determine the client's communication and learning system.

2. To discuss what hypnosis is and is not to include the elimination of fears and misconceptions the client may have about hypnosis.
3. To learn the client's motivation so that you can formulate effective suggestions.
4. To prepare the client for the induction through suggestibility exercise.
5. Induction and therapy. The clinical interview and pre-talk is also a time for you to further establish yourself with your client as an expert hypnotherapist. If your client believes that you can help him achieve his goals, in all likelihood you can. He will succeed if he expects to. Therefore, you must be at your professional best, maintaining control during the interview while showing your sincere desire to help him. The person who expects to respond to hypnosis usually does so.

(4) Guidelines for Structuring Suggestions

1. Use present tense: Construct your suggestions as if they have already been accomplished or being accomplished. "You are a non-smoker. Your self-confidence is increasing more and more each and every day." Even future behavior is given in the present tense. "Next Thursday when you speak at the banquet, you are calm, relaxed, and confident." When dealing with a physical condition such as a broken leg the progressive form of the present tense is used to bypass the critical factor of the conscious mind. "Each day your leg is healing faster and faster. Your leg is becoming stronger and stronger."

   Using the word "will" reduces the effectiveness of the suggestion because it is indefinite. Any suggestion given in the future tense with the word, "will" is like making a New Years's resolution.

2. Use positive instead of negative statements as the subconscious mind may drop the "not" or "no" and accept the suggestions opposite to the desired meaning. For example: If someone who wants to remain awake and alert while driving a car, says, "I will not get sleepy while driving." If the subconscious mind drops the "not," what has the subconscious

heard? A better suggestion would be: "While I am driving, I will remain awake and alert."

3. Do not use the word "try." "Try" implies failure. Someone said to me, "I tried to call you last night." Well, either he picked up the phone, dialed my number and got a busy signal or no answer or he did not call at all. If the person dialed my number and got a busy signal or no answer, he did not try to call me, he called me, he just did not make contact with me. "Try to pick up a cup of coffee." You either pick it up or you let it sit there.

   In the *Star Wars* movie, "The Empire Strikes Back," Yoda tells Luke to levitate his space ship out of a swap by thought alone. Luke says, "OK, I will try." Yoda responds, "Try not, do, do, or do not. There is no try." Though Luke makes the attempt, he's unsuccessful. After much effort, he says, "I can't. It's too big." Yoda then raises his arm, closes his eyes, and raises spacecraft from the swamp and sets it on dry land. Luke says, "I don't believe it." Yoda quickly replies, "That is why you failed."

4. Imagine or visualize what you want to happen as if it has already happened.

5. Be specific. Choose one area to work on at a time or a few related areas. You can work with improving self-confidence with about anything you are working on. You can work on a few related issues, but too many may become confusing to the subconscious mind. If the client wants to cover two areas, ask which one is more important and work on that issue first. Example: If the person comes for stop smoking and weight control. I recommend that you work with client for stop smoking first with a few weight control suggestions included. The reason I make this recommendation is that stopping smoking is usually easier to overcome.

6. Be detailed. Analyze the goal and structure your suggestions to cover details of the changed behavior and/or attitude.

7. Be simple. Speak to the subconscious as you would a bright 9-year-old. In most cases avoid long technical terms.

8. Use exciting words: joyous, radiant, thrilling, abundant, loving, wonderful.

9. When a suggestion is coupled with an emotion, the suggestion is enhanced.

10. Be accurate: name exactly what the client desires to achieve. "You reduce to your desire weight to 125 lbs."

11. Be realistic. To suggest that a 57-year-old man can be a major league ballplayer may be unrealistic. If the individual involved is capable, you may suggest he consider a softball league or a senior baseball league.

12. Personalize the suggestion. Take information obtained in the interview and integrate the clients concerns into the script you use with the client.

13. Be repetitive. Repeat the suggestion, repeat the suggestion, repeat the suggestion. Repetition is important because it helps to strengthen the suggestion and aid in its retention. It may be helpful to repeat the suggestion several times with a slight change in wording. Example: "You are satisfied with just enough food to meet your body's nutritional needs, you are satisfied with just enough food to meet your body's nutritional needs, you are satisfied with just enough food to meet your body's nutritional needs. You find that you feel full with small portions of healthy food. You enjoy the feeling of eating good food in limited quantities."

(5) Types of Suggestions

1. Direct Suggestions are to the point and request desired results, "You desire those foods which help you reach your goal." "You have been released from your desire to smoke."

2. Indirect Suggestions relates to the situation you are working with, but in covert ways. Indirect suggestions tend to give the impression of choice. "Are you gaining self-confidence because I suggest it or because you are learning to be more confident." The implied meaning is that the individual is becoming more confident. "Have you made the decision to be a non-smoker because you want to be healthier or because you want to use the money saved on other things?"

3. Open-Ended Suggestions are designed to be interpreted in the broadest manner possible as a means to enhance the ben-

efits of trance. In the initial stages of trance, the suggestion, "There are many ways of finding the most comfortable position conductive to trance," is an example of the open-ended suggestion.

"You may find yourself reviewing and remembering these things you learned in trance for some time to come."

"Imagine yourself as a non-smoker, act as if you are a non-smoker and you are a non-smoker because . . ."

4. Positive Suggestions are used because the subconscious mind tends to respond better to positive suggestion. "When you are driving, you remain awake and alert." Instead of "When you are driving you will not get sleepy." If the subconscious mind doesn't pick up the "not," what has your subconscious mind accepted?

5. Negative Suggestions uses words like "no," "not," as in the above suggestion about "not going to sleep" while driving a car. Negative suggestions can be given as a type of reverse psychology. If I were to say to you, "Do not think of the number seven." What do you do? You can't help but think of the number seven. "Do not think about how deep you are going, just go deeper."

6. Truisms are statements which are generally regarded as true and they are used to develop an attitude of acceptance of the statement that follows. "As two plus two is four, and as you breathe in and out, you go into a deeper and deeper state of hypnosis."

   "The subconscious part of your mind is an amazing storehouse of memories that enables you to go into a deep hypnotic state . . . to find out numerous things you can do . . . and you are capable of doing much more than you have ever been aware of . . . "

   By using truisms, you are giving indirect suggestions of things the person is familiar with or knows to be true and these can be associated with the response you are wanting the client to experience.

7. Suggestions Covering All Possible Alternatives such as "As you allow your arms to relax, you may notice that your arms

and hands feel pleasantly light or comfortably heavy, or maybe you are just more aware of your hands than you were before I mentioned them."

"You may find yourself going into trance slowly or quickly, now or later. You may choose to release this problem now, later today, or tomorrow." Implication is that problem will be released.

In addition to those people who are direct and indirect suggestible, there is a third class, which may show up as direct or indirect, but are classified as analytical. These people analyze or question whatever you may say. Suggestions which use all possible alternatives are good for analytical because they cover all possibilities of response. With these suggestions, any response is correct, including no response at all.

A suggestion which covers all possible alternatives may go something like this: "As I count from ten down to one, you may find your right hand moving, or perhaps it may be your left hand that moves. . . . It may move up or it may press down more tightly against your thigh, or it may move to the side. It may move quickly or slowly . . . or it may begin jerking, or perhaps it may not move at all. It is not important the way your hand moves, the important thing is to be fully aware of the feelings that develop . . . as you go deeper and deeper."

The various possibilities of hand movement are covered, including the possibility of not moving at all. Using this type of suggestion during the induction, there is no way for the client to fail. He is successful regardless of what response may develop.

By using this type of induction, it gives you a chance to observe what type of responsiveness that particular client is achieving. At the same time, you are inducing the hypnotic trance by getting his conscious mind to focus on his hand or hands instead of questioning what is happening.

8. Permissive Suggestions are suggestions which are requested for the client to follow. "You may want to close your eyes as you allow yourself to relax more and more."
9. Apposition of opposites is the technique which involves the use of opposing behavior or states. "You may find yourself feeling

lighter as you go deeper into trance." In age regression, one may say, "The older you become, the younger your memories may be." Using contradictory messages are more likely to promote confusion that can help the suggestions to by-pass the critical factor of the conscious mind and the enter the subconscious mind where it can be acted upon for change.

10. Binds of Comparable Alternatives are statements that offer the client a free choice of two or more comparable alternatives that may lead to more constructive behavior . . . "Would you prefer to use your right hand or your left hand to respond." "You can choose how you use this trance or may simply discover its use."

11. Double Blinds are presented at the conscious level to effect change in the subconscious. The double bind offers alternative choices in order to counter a negative response. If you ask a person, "Would like a soft drink?" It is easy to say, "no," but not easy if you say, "Would you prefer a Coke or a Dr. Pepper or maybe a Pepsi either diet or regular?" Another example of a double bind is, "You think you know the real reasoning behind your problem, but maybe your subconscious sees things differently. Maybe your conscious understands imperfectly what your subconscious understands perfectly. Whereas your conscious mind may be confused, your subconscious mind can now move toward the resolution of the problem."

    "Maybe your conscious mind can give you permission to go into trance while your subconscious mind prepares for change or maybe your subconscious mind triggers your willingness to enter trance while your conscious mind gets ready to receive new information and understanding."

    For a resistant client: "I don't want you to listen to me even if you feel like you want to relax and pay attention. I am positive that there is nothing that I say that can be of any use to you, so don't even try to absorb any of this information." This technique averts the client's attention as he begins to wonder what is going on as you continue with good positive suggestions for the subconscious.

    "You can either go into trance as we speak, or you can begin to notice changes in your consciousness and experiences." The client has a choice, and both are beneficial to the client.

12. Compounding The Suggestions occurs when you tie a suggestion to a specific pattern or behavior. "As you continue breathing deeply and slowly, you keep becoming more and more relaxed and comfortable." The client is breathing, so you associate relaxation and comfort to breathing deeply and slowly.

    "As you continue sitting there, you keep drifting into a deeper and deeper hypnotic state."

    "In a moment I am going to ask you to open your eyes and remain in hypnosis. I will ask you to move over to that other chair and when you are comfortable in that other chair, I will ask you to close your eyes. When you close your eyes, you will go twice as deep into hypnosis."

13. "If" and "Then": These two by-words can be tremendously effective when inserted into a sentence properly. "If you learn to use these two key words in the right way and at the right times then you increase the effectiveness of your suggestions 100%."

    "If you close your eyes for a couple minutes each night and imagine your body the way you want it to be, then your subconscious mind causes it to happen, and you develop a perfect body, exactly the way you want it to be."

14. Aversion Suggestions are used to change behavior by making it have a negative effect upon the client. "Your cigarettes taste like horse manure." I seldom use aversion suggestions because I prefer positive change in behavior. "Chocolate candy taste like gummy tar. You want to spit it out because it taste so bad." "You are trying to get heavy phlegm out of your throat caused by smoking. Will it be slimy green or yellow? Will it have blood in it? Feel yourself gagging to bring it up . . . It will disappear when you are a non-smoker." I would never use such a suggestion. The only time I have ever used aversion suggestions was when a man came back for a third session. He said, "Tell me my cigarettes taste awful." I followed his request and he stopped smoking. It worked for him because that was the kind of suggestions he expected. His uncle had quit smoking and had always told him that is the way hypnosis worked.

15. Metaphor and Healing Stories are indirect methods of suggestion. They are stories which point to some meaning beyond the

story so that the client can use them to motivate change. They are non-threatening to the client and are available to the client to discover its therapeutic meaning for himself.

(6) Types of Imagery

1. Spontaneous Imagery comes to one without consciously requesting the imagery. I can remember a time while visiting the pastor of Arcadia Methodist Church—as I drove by the old Joy Theater (still standing, but not in use) I could almost see myself as a 5- to 9-year-old boy going to that theater. It was usually on a Saturday afternoon and a double feature western was the order of the day. What a good time I had in my spontaneous age regression.

2. Induced Imagery is consciously selected for a specific purpose. One day, as I was thinking of my dad who died in 1983, I consciously went back in my mind to the night before I went to college. I could see my dad plainly as he said to me, "Paul, you are going to be taught many things while in college. Some will be different from what you have been taught at home. Take that which will help you whether it is like you have been taught or not and add it to your life. If it does not help, discard it." He continued to talk and finished his guidance with these words, "Be careful what you pray for and what you preach against, because you might get them both."

   I did not have to ask my dad what he meant. I understand him to mean, "If you pray to miss an event that you do not want to attend, you may get sick and not have to attend." The prayer was answered but the person did not want to get sick. In regards to the preaching statement, he meant often that which one is against, may be the biggest temptation for that individual. One who preaches against the "sins of the flesh" may get into trouble by having sex outside of marriage.

3. Concrete imagery is used to see something in detail which you want to happen in your life. A person who desires to reduce to a specific weight uses an imagery of stepping on the scales and seeing the exact weight she desires to be.

4. Abstract imagery has the person in number 3, seeing a bowl of ice cream behind a red circle with a red bar crossing the bowl. That is the universal symbol for "reframe from."
5. General imagery is used to see yourself healthy, feeling good, enjoying life. This imagery is used for overall achievement instead of specific results.
6. Specific imagery is used for a specific purpose. A person with high blood pressure imagines taking his blood pressure and seeing 120 over 80.
7. End Results imagery is used to imagine the end result which is desired. I have shared with you the imagery that I used before being selected for promotion to Brigadier General. I visualized my star being pinned on me by the Chief of Chaplain of the Army and wearing my general's uniform.
8. Process imagery is used in going through a process by which the goal is achieved. A person in preparation for a speech imagines preparing the speech, choosing just the right things to say, writing the speech, practicing the speech, and delivering the speech.
9. Guided imagery is scripted to bring about a specific imagery. "Imagine that you are walking down a beautiful country road. It is a beautiful sunny day . . . "

Section Three

Case Histories

Chapter Nineteen
Hypnosis with Children

Though children are considered very responsive to the hypnotic state, there is very little written on the subject. Two or three books and a few articles have been published over the last few years, but this is an area where more information is needed.

Except for a few hypnotherapists throughout the nation who specialize in children hypnotherapy, most of the rest of us seldom work with children. I occasionally work with children and have discovered it to be a challenge. I do not write this chapter as an expert in the field of children hypnotherapy but to share with you an experience of working with a child.

Most children over five years old have the necessary verbal understanding to be hypnotized, but even younger children can be hypnotized. Could not the rocking of a baby, singing to a baby, softly talking to a baby be considered hypnotic techniques? Most children have a vivid and active imagination which makes them very susceptible to suggestion. Using the child's natural tendency to pretend and make-believe enhances the use of hypnosis with children. Children tend to have short attention spans and this should be kept in mind when working with a child.

Induction methods and induction talks will vary with the age of the child. It is important to talk on a level which the child can understand. A small child may not know what the word "relax" means but can be told to make a tight fist and let it go to demonstrate relaxation. The child can be told to let his muscles become loose and floppy.

For the best induction, find something the child is interested in, perhaps a TV show, space travel, or heroes. Tell the child that you want to tell them a story and it may be more interesting with the eyes closed. Do not demand eye closure because this may interfere with the induction. In the story, use the child's favorite place, hero, TV show, etc.

One should never use "baby talk," "speak over their head," or "talk down to the child." There should be no unexpected change in tone or content.

Hypnotherapy has been effective for helping children overcome bed wetting, nail-biting, phobias, stammering, asthma, tics, and behavioral problems associated with tension, stress and other difficulties. Compared to adults, children are more physically active, more likely to open their eyes to refuse to shut them, and more likely to speak spontaneously during hypnosis.

Words like "sleep," "tired," and "drowsy" should be avoided because many children have negative altitudes about sleep. What if the child had a pet who got sick and the child's parent said they were going to have "Bobo" put to sleep. The parents return but Bobo doesn't. The child then may associate the "sleep" with death or abandonment.

(1) Ned with the School Phobia Case History

Ten year-old Ned's mother called me regarding her son's school phobia. He hated to go to school and would leave school at his first chance and return home. Over the last several weeks, Ned had not spent an entire day at school. He was seeing a psychologist so I requested that the parents have the psychologist consult me, and I would work with Ned. The psychologist who was working with Ned was a friend and we often referred clients to each other. The next day I received the consult so I called Ned's parents and an appointment was scheduled for the next Friday.

Ned lived in Mississippi, about an hour's drive to New Orleans. Both mother and father accompanied Ned to the session. While Ned and his father filled out the counseling information paper, I talked with Ned's mother. Ned did not want to come, had cried since they had left home and was very upset. His mother told me that he was afraid that he would be admitted to the hospital. On a previous visit to another hospital in New Orleans, Ned had been admitted. Following the hospitalization, there was little or no change in his fear of school.

When I finished talking to Ned's mother, we walked out of my office into the reception room. I told Ned that he could have either or both of his parents and that we would not do hypnosis without his consent. Ned asked his dad to come into my office with him.

Once in the office, I said to Ned, "You don't want to be here, do you?" "No sir." "I can understand you not wanting to be here for you are uncertain what will happen. I can assure you that you will not be admitted to the hospital and you will return to Mississippi with your parents today. I want to talk to you and explain something about hypnosis so that you can see that it will be a very pleasant experience." He said, "OK."

"First, I would like for you to tell me in your own words why you are here today." He told a story similar to his mother's account. I asked him if he liked his teachers and he said they were OK. I asked him if he had any trouble with any student which contributed to his fear of school. He said two years ago, one student scared him and he was afraid to go to school but had gotten over it. That student was not even in his school now.

I asked him if I could show him something and he said, "yes." I picked up a paper sack from my desk drawer. I removed a block of wood with a nail standing in the middle of the block and six more nails.

I asked Ned if he thought I could balance all those nails on the one standing in the middle of the block. I told him that I could not tie them together nor magnetize them so they would stick together. Ned did not think I could balance the nails. I put them together in the appropriate manner, picked up the nails and they balanced on top of the nail in the block. Ned was impressed. I concluded the balancing act with the statement, "As I could balance the nails which looked impossible, you can learn to do something which seems impossible to you now such as going to and staying in school."

(2) The Wizard of Oz (adapted from Krasner)

As *The Wizard of Oz* had been on TV a few nights before, I asked if he had seen it on TV and he said, "Yes." I told him this story adapted form book, *The Wizard Within* by Dr. A.M. Krasner.

The first time I saw *The Wizard of Oz,* I was in the seventh grade in Avenger, Texas. Classes were dismissed and our class went to see the movie. I guess I enjoyed that movie most of all because we got out of school a half day to see *The Wizard of Oz*. I have seen it several times on TV since that time and always seem to experience some new or additional meaning.

Each major character in *The Wizard of Oz* carries with it a message. The grand and mighty Wizard turns out to be just a common man who guides the character to the solutions they hold within themselves. The Wicked Witch of the West whom Dorothy and her companions flee in terror, turns out to be defeat with a bucket of water. The problem that each character brings to the Wizard turns out to be something each already had. The Lion always had courage, the Scarecrow had a brain, the Tin Man always had a heart and Dorothy always had the ability to get back home. Their problem was they did not realize their abilities until the Wizard helped them discover their capabilities.

You remember the story of Dorothy and her dog Toto. They made the perilous journey along the Yellow Brick Road with their companions the Cowardly Lion, the Tin Woodsman and the Scarecrow. The unlikely group went through many exciting adventures and frightening experiences in order to reach the Land of Oz where the Wizard lived. They believe that he—and only he—could grant their wishes.

The scarecrow wanted a brain. The Tin Woodsman wanted a heart. The Lion wanted courage. Of course, the three of them already had these things, but they didn't believe they did. After stuffing the Scarecrow's head with a combination of things the Wizard of Oz declared, "I have given you brains. Hereafter you will be a great man." The Scarecrow believed the Wizard and he felt wise indeed. The Wizard took a silk heart filled with sawdust and placed it in the Tin Woodsman's breast. The Wizard said, "Now, you have a heart any man would be proud of." The Tin Woodsman believed the Wizard and felt tender and loving. The Lion drank a special potion which, according to the Wizard was courage. "Drink this," said the Wizard, "And you will be filled with courage." Believing the Wizard, the Lion drank the potion and feared nothing. Never mind that the Wizard turned out to be an ordinary man, he was extraordinary in that he had the capacity to engender belief. He helped change the course of people's lives by changing their beliefs about themselves.

During the course of the story, the Scarecrow was brilliant, the Tin Woodsman was kind and helpful and the Lion was fearlessly courageous. They knew they could do things . . . The Wizard of Oz had told them so and they believed him. You have within you the solution to your fear of going to school and you can release those fears if you believe you can.

Instead of tears running down his face, there was now a smile. I talked to him about hypnosis being a very relaxing experience and that he could use his imagination to help him make changes in his life which he desired. I asked him if he would do an experiment with me and he said he would like that. I did "Taste the Lemon" exercise and "Hand Heavy, Hand Light" exercise. He was impressed with the results of these exercises so I asked him to close his eyes and he did. I asked him to open his eyes and he did. I asked him to stand up and he did. I asked him to stand on his head and he looked at me as if I was crazy. I quickly said, "And you would not stand on your head if you had been in hypnosis. You followed my suggestion until I gave one that seemed foolish to you. The same is true when you are in hypnosis."

I asked him if he was willing to use hypnosis to help him overcome his fear and he said, "Yes."

His mother told me that he liked going on boat rides with his dad in the canal near their home. I asked him if he would like to go on an imaginary boat ride with his dad and he nodded, "Yes." I told him he could keep his eyes open or he could shut them. He closed his eyes. I developed an imagery of the boat ride and he felt tired so he could lie down in the boat because his dad would be keeping the boat on course. I proceeded with a progressive relaxation technique using the movement of the boat for deepening.

I followed with a desensitization exercise by having him lift a finger at the first feeling of fear, then taking deep breath and blowing the fear out as he exhaled. I went step by step from waking up in the morning, getting dressed, going to school, walking to the school house door, going to his room, teacher beginning class, and went through the school day. I went over each area until there was no finger signal of fear and then went to the next activity. I went back over the entire procedure beginning with his getting up in the morning till he returned home from school with no finger signal for fear.

(3) The Green Dragon (adapted from Wallas' *Stories For The Third Ear*)

I use this with most clients with a phobia regardless of age.

Once upon a time there was a little boy (or girl, depending on the client) who was very, very rich. He was so rich that he had a large room just for his toys and treasurers. He went to his toy room just about every day. Now you would think that he would be very, very happy little boy because he had so many toys, but such was not the case.

Actually, the little boy was very, very sad because although he had many toys, there was one thing that spoiled everything for him. Sitting over in the corner of the room, barely visible behind all the heaped-up toys, sat a large, green dragon. This dragon never seemed to take its eyes off the little boy.

No matter what the little boy was doing, whenever he looked up, there was the green dragon watching him. This would spoil his fun, for he was very much afraid of the dragon. He would think to himself that the green dragon may someday attack him, throw him down on the floor and harm him. As a result of worrying about the green dragon, he felt very, very unhappy.

Some days he would dance and play very hard; he would whirl around, laugh very loud, and talk a blue streak in hopes that he could forget about the dragon in the corner. No matter how loudly he laughed, how hard he played or how fast he danced and whirled and jumped, when he stopped, he would look in the corner and there wold be the green dragon still staring and looking very, very dangerous. The little boy would sit down feeling fear and defeat. His fun was spoiled again by the presence of the green dragon. Each day, the little boy would begin the day playing with his toys, happily trying to forget about the green dragon, and each day he would end the day sitting quiet and sad with tears running down his face.

One day, a friend came to visit the boy. The friend was a boy about his age and size. The friend looked around the room with his eyes opening wider and wider and said, "Oh, what wonderful toys!" He ran around picking up this one and that one and playing and clapping his hands, but the little rich boy felt anxious and worried. He kept glancing at the green dragon.

Suddenly, to his horror, he saw his friend run over to the green dragon and started to sit astride the dragon's back. The little boy cried, "No, don't do that!" His friend responded, "Why not? this is fun!" The little boy said, "He is such a fierce and ugly dragon. Surely, he will harm you. I am so afraid of him."

"Ho, ho, ho," said his friend, "Look at this." He turned the dragon so the little boy could see, and down the back of the dragon was a long, shiny zipper. The little boy did not know what to make of it. He watched with eyes wide open, still trembling with fear. The friend said, "Shall I unzip it?" The little boy replied, "I'm not sure. I am afraid." His friend said, "Nonsense!" and unzipped the dragon. When he did, the green dragon suit fell down. What do you think was there? The little rich boy himself or rather that part of him that was so afraid of what he did not understand. The little boy realized that the green dragon was just an extension of himself. He had been afraid of his own fears.

The little boy began to laugh and his friend joined him in his laughter. The little boy could laugh because he realized that now he was free from his fear of the green dragon. Now he was happy. He played with his toys and shared them with his friend. Soon he had other friends visit him and they enjoyed the toys. He realized that he no longer needed to be afraid of the dragon because he had come to understand his fears and release them.

Now I wonder if you might feel a smile coming over your face today as you release your fears. You have slain your dragon and have released your fears and if it is so, you began to smile. You may try to hold the smile back but the harder you try, the bigger the smile becomes. Ned began to smile. I gave him some self-confidence suggestions and said that he would experience a cycle of progress as day-by-day he had more and more confidence in himself. I then counted him out of the hypnotic state and he felt very good about himself. He asked, "If I need to, can I come back to see you?" and I responded, "Yes, of course."

Chapter Twenty
Stop Smoking

The most popular known and best advertised use of hypnosis is for habit control. Perhaps stop smoking heads the list of those habits that respond favorably to hypnosis. People who come to a hypnotherapist with the desire to stop smoking comes for a variety of reasons, different degrees of motivation and mixed feelings or desires.

When motivated and an individual's desire to stop smoking is genuine, breaking the habit with hypnosis is relatively simple. I have had individuals come in my office and say, "Hypnotize me and make me stop smoking." I respond, "I cannot make you do anything. If you are ready to stop smoking, I can help you, but I can't make you stop."

After being paged to come to the Intensive Care Unit (ICU), I was told by the nurse that Mr. Mann had said that he was going to smoke a cigarette, even if he had to pull out his IV's and leave the hospital. The nurse asked me if I would go in and calm him down. When I entered the room, Mr. Mann said, "I came to you to stop smoking five years ago." I responded, "What happened? Did you start smoking again?" He said, "No, I never quit, but it was not your fault. I was smoking six packs of cigarettes a day and since then I have smoked only six cigarettes a day. You see my wife nagged me so much and for so long to quit smoking that I was not going to give her the satisfaction of knowing she won so I continued to smoke those six cigarettes a day. This is why I want one now."

We talked for about ten minutes and I said, "You do not have to do without a cigarette because your wife wants you too. For your health and well being, you can choose to cease smoking until you go home. Of course, since it would be your own decision and not someone elses, you may choose to quit smoking even after you get out of the hospital." I do not know what happened after Mr. Mann got out of the hospital, but at least he chose not to smoke while he was in the hospital.

When a person is properly motivated, it generally takes only one session. In fact, I tell the client that I do not think it will be needed, but she/he can return any time within the next 30 days for a follow-up at no extra cost.

As with any situation, I go over what hypnosis is and what it is not, how hypnosis can help the person become a non-smoker in the easiest possible way. I emphasize the characteristic of the subconscious mind to keep in process anything that has developed into a habit. I agree with the former Surgeon General that smoking is a difficult habit to overcome, but it is not because of the nicotine habit, but because of the subconscious effect to keep the habit going. Only a very small percent of people have a hard nicotine habit. The low success rate of the patch verify what I am saying.

(1) John's Case History

John was a thirty-year-old man who came to me for help in overcoming his smoking habit. As I do with all clients, I went over with him the basic pre-talk concerning hypnosis and how it can help him be a nonsmoker. During the first session, I ask these questions of John (and others who come for stop smoking hypnosis): How long have you been smoking? "15 years." Have you ever stopped smoking in the past? "Yes, I quit for about six months following surgery. That must have been about three years ago." Why did you start again?

"My mother died and at the wake, some of my friends and family were smoking so I asked for one and I was back to being a smoker." Do you wake up during the night to smoke? "No." Good, that means your habit is primarily a psychological habit. (If "yes," I put a greater emphasis on releasing nicotine from the body and sleeping through the night.)

I am going to ask you some questions which can be answered *Yes* or *No*. Do you smoke when you feel lonely? *Yes*. Tired? *Yes*. Bored? *Yes*. Stressed? *Yes*. Insecure? *Yes*. Awkward? *Yes*. Uncomfortable? *Yes*. Angry or upset? *Yes*. Do you smoke before breakfast? *No*. In your car? *Yes*. While watching TV? *Yes*. After meals? *Yes*. At work? *No*. Talking on the phone? *Yes*. In bed? *No*. While reading? *No*. With coffee? *Yes*. At social events? *Depends on whether smoking is allowed or not*. Do you smoke when you need companionship? *Yes*. A break in routine? *Yes*. Comfort? *No*. Relaxation? *Yes*. To control desires? *No*. In place of food? *No*. To be noticed? *No*. To look occupied? *No*.

Is there anything that triggers a smoke? "Yes, I tend to light up when I get in my car, talk on the phone, or drink a cup of coffee except at the office." How many cigarettes do you smoke a day? "20." Why do you want to stop smoking? "For my health, I don't like the cough I have when I wake up in the morning. I play in a softball league and want to breath easier and exercise with more comfort." After the pre-talk, questions, and induction, I began the therapy.

(2) You Can Be a Non-Smoker

You have decided to stop smoking. This is your own decision. You are doing this for your own benefit, and for your own well being. You are doing this because you want to be healthier, you want to breath easier and be more comfortable while exercising and playing softball. This means it is easy for you to get rid of the smoking habit through hypnosis.

In fact, you have already stopped smoking, because you are realizing how calm and relaxed you are right now, even though you don't have a cigarette in your hand or mouth. This relaxation that you are experiencing is a very peaceful, calm state which you produced yourself. In the same way you became calm and relaxed every time you take a good deep breath and exhale. As you breathe out, tension leaves your body and a calm relaxed state takes over. Now, Let your memory carry you back in time when you accomplished something that brought you a sense of pride and well being. It can be something that happened recently or something that happened years ago. It can be something you did for yourself or something you did for someone else. It can be a mission accomplished or a goal attained. When you have the memory in your awareness, nod your head, "Yes." Thank you, now allow yourself to feel that pride and well-being as completely as you can: physically, emotionally, spiritually.

Now anchor that feeling by touching the first finger and thumb of the hand in which you normally hold a cigarette. Now, whenever you have a desire for a cigarette, take a good deep breath, touch the first finger and thumb together and as you exhale, the need and desire for that cigarette leaves your mind and body and in its place comes a sense of pride, accomplishment and peace.

You know that you need food to provide your body with proper nourishment but you eat at the appropriate time and the appropriate amount. You refuse to exchange an eating habit for a smoking habit. You feel good about yourself and you can maintain your current weight. You need water for proper body maintenance, but there is nothing in a cigarette which your body needs. Each hour, each day, each week, every month you go as a non-smoker your lungs get cleaner, healthier, pinker . . . Your heart functions more normally because it no longer has to pump the extra weight of nicotine and tar through your body. Your circulatory system functions more properly because it no longer has to carry the extra weight of nicotine and tar throughout your body. Day by day in every way you are getting healthier and healthier as a non-smoker. (For "Stop Smoking" I usually use the "Walk In The Country: Heavy Backpack" imagery at this point in the session. However, I will use that imagery with "Weight Control." For this session, I will use "Free from Jail.")

(3) Free from Jail

You find yourself in a jail cell and you are behind bars. As you look at the bars in the window, each bar looks like a cigarette. As you look at the bars on the door, they look like king-size cigarettes. As you look about the jail cell, you realize that you are in a jail cell of your own making. You notice a key in the lock of the door. If you want to be free of your conscious and subconscious need to smoke, allow one of your fingers to rise indicating that you have made a decision to unlock the prison cell and be free. If you are ready to be free from the conscious and subconscious need to smoke, turn the key, unlock the door, be free and allow one of your fingers to rise. (The finger rises.) There it is, you have been set free from the conscious and subconscious need to smoke. You are free from the smoking habit. In the past cigarettes have controlled your, now you are in control. Now let your finger float back down to your lap, as you go deeper and deeper.

You have stopped smoking completely, and your subconscious mind is now working for you by causing your body processes to function properly to cleanse all nicotine, tar, and all other impurities caused by smoking, rapidly from your body. All desires to smoke are leaving your mind and body. As your subconscious assists you, your will-power and self-control are becoming stronger every hour, enabling you to be completely free from the smoking habit.

You are calm and relaxed even when you are around other people who are smoking. You are calm and relaxed. When you see other people smoking, it makes you happy that you are a non-smoker. You are proud of the fact that you are a non-smoker.

Tobacco loses its appeal to you. You may be able to enjoy the smell of tobacco when someone else is smoking, but you have been released from the desire to smoke yourself. You have quit smoking completely. You have been completely released from the smoking habit. You are happy to feel the freedom you now enjoy. You feel like a great load has been lifted from you. All desire for smoking is being cleansed out of your body completely.

(4) CRUTCHES

There was a man (or woman, depending on the sex of the client) who lived in a strange country. Now, this was a strange country because most of the adults walked with crutches even though they had no physical handicap requiring crutches. It just seemed the thing to do and most teenagers started using crutches because it seemed to be the mature thing to do and most of their peers used crutches.

Now there were disadvantages to using crutches. They slowed the person down and caused them to interfere with the safety of others as they might bump into another or accidentally trip another person.

One day this man was walking several blocks from his home, he found the little boy who lived next door to him. The little boy, who was about three years old, was by himself and he was crying. He apparently had wandered away from home and was lost. Without thinking, the man dropped his crutches, took the little boy and walked him home. The mother was overjoyed that her son was home and the little boy was happy. Later that night, the man all of sudden remembered that he had left his crutches on the street where he had found the little boy. His first thought was to run down the street to see if he could find his crutches. If not, he could go to a convenience store and buy a new pack. The man said to himself, "I have gone without my crutches this long, I can go without them the rest of my life." He did, and so can you.

Each hour you keep feeling healthier and healthier, stronger and stronger, cleaner and cleaner. Imagine yourself going through the day without a cigarette and feeling good about your accomplishment. Whenever you get in your car, you are reminded of how happy you are to be a non-smoker. Whenever you pick up the phone, you are reminded of how glad you are to be a non-smoker. Whenever you pick up a cup of coffee, you enjoy the aroma and the taste for you experience the full flavor of the coffee and you are proud to be a non-smoker. As you play softball, you breath easier and you are more comfortable. It is good to start the day breathing easy and freely. It is good to be free of the smoking habit.

At the count of three, you come out of this hypnotic experience knowing that you have a valuable tool to help you be a non-smoker. One, Whenever you have a desire to smoke or feel stressed, just take a good deep breath, touch the first finger and thumb of your right hand and as you exhale, the need and desire for a smoke leaves if or mind and body and you have a feeling of pride, accomplishment, and peace. Two, you come out feeling that you have had an hour of energy restoring sleep, but it in no way affects your ability to sleep tonight. In fact, you sleep better tonight than you have in a long time. Coming out feeling confident in yourself as a non-smoker. Three.

Very few clients have to come back for a second session, but I chose John's case because he did need a second session. He returned about two weeks later for his second session. He explained, "I was doing OK until two nights ago. I got mad at my girl friend and so I smoked a cigarette. One cigarette lead to another so that's why I am back."

(5) Stop Smoking #2

As you are relaxed and comfortable, you are now ready to allow your subconscious mind to make some pleasant changes within you so that you change from being a smoker to being a non-smoker. In fact, your subconscious mind is already directing your natural body processes to eliminate all nicotine, tar and other impurities caused by smoking from your sinuses, from your throat, from your lungs, from your blood, and from the rest of your body through your normal elimination systems.

You have accepted the responsibility for taking care of your own body. By having this session, you have made a commitment to protect your body from now on by deciding to never smoke again. You have made a wise decision. You are now in control and you are a non-smoker because you are dissatisfied with the way smoking affects you. I am suggesting to your subconscious mind that you need your body to live and you want to live the rest of your life in a healthy body, so you are determined that you have stopped smoking for your health and well being.

Now that you are a non-smoker, you know your body is healthier and stronger. You'll find that you feel much better now that you have discontinued the smoking habit. This is your own decision. You have ceased smoking for your own benefit, for your own personal well being, for your own health, and for others as well (list other reasons client came for stop smoking).

You are happy to notice how much better you feel now that you are a non-smoker. You are happy to know that your subconscious mind has already started the process of cleansing the nicotine, tar, and other impurities out of your body through normal functions of your eliminations systems. When you come out of this hypnotic state, you release all desire for smoking. All desire to smoke is leaving.

You are happy to find that your will-power and self-control keep increasing, more and more each hour. You have stopped smoking already. You realize that you are peaceful and calm right now, even though you don't have a cigarette in your hand or mouth, nor do you have one burning in an ash tray. Remember that you have a signal to help you whenever you have a desire to smoke or when you feel a need to be calm as you go about your daily activities. The signal is simple: take a good deep breath, touch the first finger and thumb together and as you exhale, the desire to smoke leaves your mind and body and you feel calm, relaxed, and you experience a sense of pride in being a non-smoker. You feel calm and relaxed. Now you have already stopped smoking, and you are in control. You know that your body needs water. Water is good for your body. It helps cleanse waste materials and impurities from your body. It helps eliminate the desire for snacks so that you maintain your present weight or even helps you to lose weight if you desire to do so.

Your body needs food to provide proteins, vitamins, minerals, fiber, potassium, and other nutrients to keep your body trim and healthy. You eat at the appropriate time and the appropriate amounts. You refuse to exchange an eating habit for a smoking habit.

Getting rid of the smoking habit causes you to have a feeling of fulfillment and gives you a strong sense of satisfaction and pride. You realize that being a non-smoker is very important to you and your health, It enables you to be an inspiration to a lot of other people who become aware of what you have accomplished.

You are already enthusiastic about your success at overcoming the smoking habit and in being a non-smoker. You are sensing a wonderful feeling of satisfaction from knowing that you are a non-smoker and you feel even better as, day by day, you become healthier and healthier.

When you are around other people who are smoking, it makes you proud that you are a non-smoker. Tobacco has lost its appeal to you. You may be able to enjoy the smell of tobacco when someone else is smoking but you are reminded by the smell (good/bad) how thankful you are to be a non-smoker.

(6) Health, Success, Motivation (for use with Stop Smoking, Weight Control, Healing)

You are now very deeply relaxed and your mind has become very receptive to the suggestions that I am giving you. I am going to ask you to think about certain words and their meaning for you. I want you to think of these words, to turn them over in your mind, to examine them, to let them sink deeply into your subconscious, as if you are planting seeds into the soil of your subconscious mind.

The first words I want you to think about are the words "good health." What can the words, "good health" mean? They can mean a sense of superb physical well-being with healthy heart and lungs; perfect functioning of all organs, nerves, glands and systems of the entire body; firm, strong muscles, bones and joints; smooth, healthy skin; increased resistance to all forms of infection or disease.

Good health can mean the body feels full of power and strength, with greater balance stamina, a greater awareness of the body, greater control of all parts of the body and a sense of harmony in the functioning of the body. Good health may mean less fatigue and illness, and proper body weight.

Good health means not only physical health, but also a healthy attitude of mind by which your nerves are calm and relaxed. The mind is calm, clear and composed. More tranquil more relaxed, more confident, more secure, and more sure of yourself. You feel better about yourself, happier and more satisfied with your life. Being a non-smoker improves your health and you are thankful you are a non-smoker.

Good health may mean that you have the ability to sleep deeply and refreshingly when you want to sleep, and then you awake feeling calm, relaxed, confident, cheerful, ready for the activity of the day with energy and enthusiasm. The words "good health" can mean all these things and more. These words have tremendous power. I want you to let them sink deeply into your subconscious mind and let them work for your good health.

The next word I would like you to think about is "success." Success may mean a sense of recognition, a fulfillment of your desires to be a non-smoker, a sense of accomplishment at being a non-smoker, an outstanding performance. It may mean a sense of worthiness and attainment of goals of being a non-smoker.

Success may mean wealthy in terms of money but it can also mean an attitude of mind which gives inner happiness and satisfaction regardless of material possessions or circumstances. I want you to use the word "success" to produce in you all the feelings that go with success.

Finally, I want you to think of the word "motivation." It can mean a gradual but progressive change in one's life; to release old recordings of negative habit patterns; to cease to fear being a puppet to one's early conditioning and to become a creator of a new, healthy, happy successful script for your life. It could mean the gradual but progressive building of a stronger and stronger feeling of self confidence and the ability to meet the challenges of life. Motivation can mean desire, determination, and a driving force to achieve a desired end of being a non-smoker. It can mean the desire to take responsibility for your own performance onto yourself, to take charge of your life and success rather than letting life's forces mold and shape your performance.

We have all been conditioned since birth to associate words with feelings. Words are therefore tools which you are going to use to produce the feeling and results which you want. These words are "good health," "success," and "motivation."

These words are used to improve health, and enable you to be more efficient and effective. This enables you to keep increasing your self-confidence, your self-esteem, your self-reliance, your self-acceptance. Each day you keep improving physically, mentally, emotionally and spiritually. You have a greater sense of your happiness that keeps increasing and you become more enthusiastic and more optimistic each day.

You are completely released from the smoking habit. You are happy to feel the freedom you now enjoy. In the past, cigarettes have controlled you, now you are in control. You feel like a big load has been lifted from you. You feel that you have been released from the prison of smoking cigarettes. You keep feeling healthier and cleaner each day. (Count out of hypnosis.)

Chapter Twenty-One
Weight Control

After introduction and same general talk about weight control, I ask, "How many times have you gone on a diet to reduce and suffered until you finally gave up without reaching your goal?" After client's answer, I say, "Perhaps you reached your goal only to gain back all that weight and added a few more pounds. Through hypnosis and self hypnosis there is help and hope."

As with any new client, I go over what hypnosis is and is not, how hypnosis helps a person to reduce and maintain their desired weight. I explain that hypnosis is not magic that can be applied with a few words of hocus-pocus and the weight magically disappears. Even with hypnosis, changing your eating habits requires some effort on the client's part.

I require at least three sessions for weight control. Of course, the client may have more if they feel that it is needed. The reasons for the three sessions to help the client maintain motivation, change eating habits, and change how they emotionally react to eating.

I require a physicians consult for weight control so that client can get proper information on appropriate foods. I do not recommend a diet, but suggest that the client select foods that will help him/her reach their goal and reject foods that would prevent them from reaching their goal. I ask the client to weigh no more than once a week, same day of week and same time.

I request that the client decide on a reasonable weight goal. I ask when was the last time you were at that weight? Do you have pictures of yourself at the desired weight? If yes, I asked the client to put one picture on the mirror where they dress each day, one on the refrigerator door, and one on the food cabinet door to remind him/her of what they have been and can be.

I talk to the client about the power of imagination and their self-image. In the past, you have come to think of yourself as heavy, overweight, and perhaps unattractive. Changing the way you think about yourself is as important as changing your eating habits. Take time each day to imagine yourself at your ideal weight. You may picture yourself before a mirror and enjoying the reflection of yourself at our desired weight. A good time to do this is just before you go to sleep each night and upon waking in the morning.

We consciously know that the beliefs which were valid for us as a child are not necessarily valid for us as an adult. But their "common sense" evaluation does not occur at the subconscious level. What was true to the subconscious yesterday is true today and will be true in the future unless we intervene to change such subconscious "truths."

For instance, a child is not eating very much food at meals. Mother and/or father says, "Now, you have to eat so that you can grow up to be a big girl/boy." If the subconscious accepts that statement from the parent, their mind may think, "I have to be big to be grown up." If a person accepts the statement with that understanding they will probably grow up to be overweight.

The first six or seven years of my life, I was skinny and sickly. At about the age of six or seven years old, I began to eat more, put on weight, and was very seldom sick. My parents and sister praised me for eating. Eating came to mean praise, reward, acceptance, and love, for me.

Those same principles are at work for many who are overweight. Though consciously the individual wants to be at the right weight for their height, she/he continues to over eat and stay fat. Perhaps their mother said, "If you are good, you may have an extra desert. Be sure to eat all the food on your plate, remember the starving children from . . ." Food comes to mean far more than nourishment. It means being loved, cared for, accepted, and rewarded.

A hypnotherapist friend of mine told me the story of a woman who came to him for weight control. She had gained 50 pounds in less than a year. After a few sessions, this story came out. She was a very religious person who was an airline stewardess. Before a flight, she and her husband had a big argument. She left the house mad and upset to go on a scheduled overseas flight. During her trip, she had an affair with one of the crew members. She felt guilty about having sex with someone other than her husband because it was against her religious belief. Her subconscious said, "I will take care of you. If you are overweight, you will not be attractive and therefore you will not be tempted to be unfaithful." With the help of her therapist, she was able to experience and accept God's forgiveness and forgive herself. With forgiveness, she was released from her need to be overweight. In less than a year, she was back to her normal weight.

(1) Deeann's Case History

Deeann came to me weighing 150 pounds. What is your desired weight? "125." During the counseling session, she told me that her husband had left her two years ago and she had gained 25 pounds since he left her. She wanted to exercise more often and eat more properly. After some finger response questions, it was determined that her weight gain was due to the stress of her divorce and she pampered herself by overeating. Her suggestibility exercises indicated that she was high in the area of direct suggestibility. She ate two meals a day with candy in between. She sometimes ate lunch but her two main meals were breakfast and dinner. With that we begin her first hypnosis session.

(2) Weight Control #1

I want you to use your imagination. Imagine that you are looking at your reflection in a mirror. Imagine yourself the size you want to be. Enjoy the experience, feel good about yourself and realize this can be you. See yourself stepping on the weight scale and weighing 125 pounds. Imagine what you want to happen so that your subconscious mind has a model to work with.

(3) Country Road: Heavy Backpack

As you relax peacefully and calmly, imagine yourself walking down a beautiful country road. To the left of the country road is a field of beautiful flowers of various colors, sizes, and shapes. If the wind is blowing just right, you can smell the fragrance of the flowers.

Beyond the flowers is a forest of majestic trees. To the right of the road is a pasture of green grass, at the foot of the pasture is a lake of blue clear water. By the lake of blue clear water are some trees, there is a stream that flows form the hill in front of you, down by the trees into the lake of blue clear water.

There is only one thing wrong with this beautiful scene. On your back is a heavy backpack. There is nothing in that backpack which you need for your journey. In fact, the backpack contains all of the conscious and subconscious reasons why you overeat, why you eat fattening foods, why you have trouble controlling our weight.

I can't remove that backpack from your back, but you can. You can be free of the heavy backpack. It is a decision for you to make. Attached to each of your fingers is a trigger mechanism which will release the backpack. If one of your fingers rises, you will release the backpack and be released from the conscious and subconscious reason why you are overweight, one of your fingers will feel very, very light, so light that it floats upwards. When the finger rises, the backpack automatically falls from your back. Now just allow one of your fingers to rise. It may be the first finger on your right hand or the first finger on your left hand, it could be the second or third, or your little finger, or it could even be the thumb. By lifting a finger, you are symbolically letting go. That is good. Your first finger of your right hand is floating up. The backpack is gone. You feel free and comfortable. As the heavy weight of the backpack is gone, you feel a great relief. You are now free of the conscious and subconscious need to be overweight.

Now that your subconscious mind is working for you, your natural body processes are eliminating unneeded and unwanted body fat through the natural processes of your elimination system. (Repeat . . . repeat . . . repeat . . .) Your confidence is increasing as you realize that you are achieving your goal of getting your body weight down to 125 pounds. (Repeat . . . repeat . . . repeat . . .)

Repeat to yourself several times, "I avoid those foods which I know are fattening." And then repeat several times, "I deserve those foods which I know helps me meet my goal." About 10 minutes before a meal, drink a large glass of water. This helps you feel full and satisfied and you are eating less food. Imagine yourself at a meal. You choose and desire those foods which help you reach your goal of 125 pounds and you refuse those foods that block your goal. Imagine picking up a fork, taking a bite of food, putting the fork down. Chew and enjoy and enjoy and chew. Get full benefit from each bite.

Visualize people complimenting you on your weight and size. As you do this each day, you reduce to 125 and you notice the improvement. This causes your confidence to keep increasing because you know you are getting your weight down to 125 pounds. As you reduce down to 125 pounds you increase your feeling of self-worth and you like yourself better. Whenever you have a desire for extra food, you can take a deep breath, imagine yourself at 125 pounds and as you exhale, the desire for that food leaves your mind as the air is breathed out. You feel calm and relaxed.

(4) Taking Off Layers

There was a young woman who lived in a very cold part of the world. It was always winter and it was always cold. The land was barren and frozen. She lived by herself and always seemed to be cold. She had a fireplace in her house, but she found it difficult to find enough wood to keep the house warm.

All of the other people in the area had moved away and she felt lonely and sad. One day there was a knock on her door. She opened the door just a crack, trying to keep the cold wind from blowing in. She peeked through the crack and asked, "Who is there?"

A woman responded, "I'm here to notify you that everyone is being evacuated from this place. You must come with me." The young woman protested, "I can't leave my house. I have nowhere to go." The stranger assured her that they would provide her with a place to live.

Fearfully, she waddled out and they started walking on a long journey.

"Where are you taking me and what will I do?" she asked, "Just trust me. I'm taking you where you will be warm and happy." But she was still fearful. They followed a path through desolate wastelands. When they had walked for several days, she noticed the landscape was changing.

She saw some shrubs and they had leaves. As they continued she began to notice some trees with leaves. One day, as they walked, she could feel moisture trickling over her body. She asked the stranger what the moisture was. The stranger told her it was sweat and told her to take off two layers of clothes. She followed the guide's suggestions and felt more comfortable, much lighter, more free, and she could walk more easily.

Each day she experienced greater delight as to how she felt. The sun was shining more, the sky was beautifully blue and she noticed that she was enjoying things that she had never noticed before. As she became warmer, she took off another layer of clothes. She felt much better and much lighter. She was able to walk faster, breathe easier, and she felt much better.

One day they arrived in a land of beautiful gardens with a beautiful lake. As she looked into the water and saw her reflection, she was pleased to notice her true self. With all but one layer of clothes gone, she saw that she was quite attractive.

She saw herself as beautiful, she felt joyful and full of energy. She felt like dancing and singing. Each day she kept feeling more free, healthier and more energetic. Her slenderness delighted her. She met other people and they told her she looked very nice. She was accepted and felt that she was part of the community.

Symbolically you are realizing that this can be your story as you get rid of layers and layers of unneeded and unwanted body fat. Everyday your self-confidence keeps increasing and your joy and happiness keeps becoming more enjoyable. Keep the image of yourself the size you want to be in your mind, eat properly, exercise appropriately, and your subconscious mind helps you reach your goal.

You reduce to 125 pounds because you look better with a slimmer body . . . You reduce to 125 pounds because it improves your health and because it helps you to live longer . . . Your reduce to 125 pounds because it helps you develop a more mature, more relaxed, more confident personality . . . You reduce to 125 pounds because it gives you the confidence to conquer any other challenging problems you face in life . . . You reduce to 125 pounds because it helps you to be an inspiration to other people who see what you have accomplished . . . You reduce to 125 pounds because it makes your life more enjoyable . . . Count out of hypnosis with helpful suggestions between each number.

During the second session, I ask these *yes* and *no* questions. Do you eat when you are hungry? *Yes.* Nervous? *Yes.* Bored? *Yes.* Stress? *Yes.* Very active? *No.* Happy? *Yes.* Lonely? *No.* Frustrated? *No.* . . . Do you eat too much or snack while watching TV? *Yes.* In groups? *Yes.* While reading? *No.* Drinking coffee? *Yes.* During breaks? *Yes.* Between work and home? *No.* At sports events? *Yes.* At social events? *Yes.* At business luncheons? *Yes.* In bed? *No.* . . . Do you treat yourself to a snack or meal whenever you need love? *Yes.* Reward? *Yes.* Companionship? *No.* Something to do? *No.* A change in your activity? *No.* To compensate for something unpleasant? *Yes.* To relax? *Yes.* To feel more important? *No.* To feel secure? *No.* In place of sexual attention? *Yes.*

(5) Selective Eating

You have a tiny gland in your brain called the appestat gland, and the purpose of that gland is to let you know when your body needs food . . . and when your body has had the right amount needed to keep you healthy and slender.

That gland is capable of functioning properly and is now being rejuvenated so it is functioning properly . . . From now on you eat only when your body needs food, and are very selective in the food you eat. That part of your mind that controls the processes of your body understands that the purpose of eating food is to provide the nourishment needed to keep your body healthy and strong . . . therefore, you select only those foods that are beneficial for your body . . . and you are perfectly content and completely satisfied with only the small amount your body needs to continue becoming healthier and remain slim and trim at the level of 125 pounds.

About ten minutes before eating you can drink a glass of water because water helps your food to digest properly. Water is also beneficial in many other ways. It aids your elimination system in functioning properly to cleanse waste products and waste materials out of your body in an easy, natural way . . . Water keeps your kidneys healthy and helps keep your urination system clean. And you can enjoy drinking lots of water.

I want you to use your imagination now . . . Imagine a very nice meal set out in front of you . . . You are dining with several close friends, and the hostess has prepared a beautiful, delicious looking meal. Look at it and notice how good it looks . . . Smell it and notice the pleasant fragrance of the food. You are looking it over and becoming aware of the small portions you can select that can benefit your body and be sufficient to take care of the needs of nourishment for your body. Now you put a small portion of those foods that are beneficial for your body on your plate, being very selective, because you eat only the right foods for your body . . . You now pick up your fork, and knife, if you need your knife, and you select the best-looking bite; remembering that the first bit is the best and most tasty because your taste buds are fresh. You put that small bite into your mouth and put your knife and fork down . . . You are chewing that bite thoroughly, really enjoying the delicious flavor of the food. Taking your time, noticing the texture, and continuing to chew the food until all the pleasurable flavor is gone, and then you swallow. You had put down your knife and fork, because you are taking your time, and now before picking it up, you take a sip of water, or tea or whatever else you are drinking with your meal. And you continue on through the entire meal, taking your time, chewing your food thoroughly and eating only until you feel satisfied and comfortable. As soon as you have eaten the small amount needed by your body, you stop, and you are satisfied. That's the way you want it to be from now on, and your inner mind is cooperating, so that's the way it can be from now on.

You eat only when your body needs food, and you eat only the small amount needed by your body at that time. When you have eaten the amount that is right to continue reducing your body and keep your body slim and trim, your are content and satisfied until your body needs food again.

You are developing the habit and pattern of eating when you are hungry, and being very selective of the foods you eat, being sure to eat only foods that are right for your body . . .

As she had expressed her grief about the divorce during the counseling session, I used "The Turning Point" healing story. (Refer to Mr. Wilder's case history in Chapter 2.)

(6) Handle for Weight Control

You may recall that the refrigerator door has a handle on it and so does the door to the food closet. Those handles can, of course, be an aid to opening those doors. The handles can also be an aid in closing the doors, but they can serve another purpose. The handle on the refrigerator door and the handle on the food closet door can be reminders to you that you have a handle on your appetite. There are times during the day when you know that opening the door to the refrigerator or food closet is appropriate when you are preparing for your regular meals . . . But during the rest of the day those door handles can represent to you an opportunity to get a better handle on yourself. You can take a look at the door handles, pause, take a deep breath to relax and imagine yourself at 125 pounds and that you have a handle of your appetite. That's right, those handles can be a constant reminder of your own control, your own handle on your goals. With that reminder, you feel good about yourself . . . (I concluded with a self-confidence script.)

When Deann came in for her third session, she was very pleased with herself. In the last three weeks, she had released eight pounds. (I am attempting to drop the word, "Lose" from my weight control program because there is a tendency to attempt to find that which is lost.)

(7) Shrinking Stomach

You are deeply relaxed and peaceful, and you can continue relaxing even more as I talk to you. You don't need to consciously listen to what I'm saying right now, because your subconscious mind, and all levels of your inner mind are receiving my words . . . and are enabling you to respond automatically. You can be pleased to find that the processes of your body are functioning properly, causing all excess cellulite and fat to dissolve and become a liquid, and is being cleansed out of your body through the normal, natural processes of your elimination system. You can also be happy to notice that you eat only small amounts of food . . . and you eat only when your body needs food. Your stomach is gradually shrinking down to the proper size to reduce your body to 125 pounds. It is normal and natural for you to eat only when your body needs food . . . and eat only the small amount your body needs to continue becoming healthier and more slender, exactly the way you consciously want your body to be.

Your self-confidence and self-acceptance keeps increasing more each day . . . Your willpower and self-control continue becoming stronger . . . and without any conscious effort by you . . . your stomach is shrinking down to the proper size to hold only the right amount of food to keep your normal, natural, 125 pound body healthy and strong. When your body needs food, you eat only the small amount needed by your body at the time . . . and when you have eaten what you body needs, you feel content, happy, and perfectly satisfied.

I want you to hold your left arm out in front of you and tighten the muscles to make your left arm stiff and rigid . . . clench your fist now and make the arm more rigid. Notice how strong and powerful it is. Feel the strong power in those muscles . . . Now, let your hand and arm relax . . . Very good. You're responding good . . . Now I want you to do it again, and this time make the fist and arm stiffer and more rigid than you did the first time . . . Make it so stiff and rigid that you can feel it aching . . . Notice that it is aching as you continue making it more rigid . . . When you have it aching so that you don't like that feeling, let it relax . . . (Pause) I want to explain something now that your mind is understanding. You make your left arm rigid and stiff two times. The actions to do that were the same each time. But the first time you did not feel any pain, because we did not sent a message to your mind for you to experience pain, but the second time as you made the arm stiff, we also sent the massage for you to experience an aching feeling. Actually it is all a matter of the way you mind interprets the signal it receives . . .

Just as easily, your stomach can send a signal to your mind, and it can happen when your stomach muscles are being stretched . . . You are learning to respond to the normal feelings of your stomach . . . When your body needs food, your stomach lets you know by causing you to feel hungry . . . When you have the hunger feeling you know it is time to eat some food to provide the proper nutrition needed by your body at that time. Then, as soon as you have eaten the proper amount needed at that time, you feel satisfied because the hunger feelings are gone until your body needs food again . . . You eat only when your stomach lets you know your body needs food . . . and you eat only the small amount needed by your body at that time. When you have eaten what your body needs at that time, you are content and satisfied, knowing your stomach lets you know when your body needs food again . . . Your stomach is shrinking because your body is reducing and you continue needing a smaller amount of food . . . You are happy to notice that your entire body is becoming more slender, trimmer, and perfectly proportioned . . . the way you consciously want it to be.

Your body is getting thinner, trimmer, and more slender, and this is just inspiring to you. It gives you a good feeling. And the fact that your stomach is shrinking just enough to reduce your body to 125 pounds and keep your body at the level of 125 pounds causes you to feel very confident and happy.

Chapter Twenty-Two

Improving Memory, Concentration, and Study Habits

Hypnosis and reinforcement by self hypnosis in improving memory and concentration is especially helpful and easy to learn and practice. Hypnosis cannot take the place of studying, reading, listening, but it can enhance the individual learning abilities and recall. Hypnosis enables the individual to tap the great resources of the subconscious mind.

There are at lease eight ways hypnosis can help improve one's scholastic abilities:

1. Increase one's ability to concentrate
2. Improve the ability to retain, recall, and remember
3. To control emotions and stress
4. Enhance motivation and enthusiasm for learning
5. Increase energy and endurance
6. Increase self-esteem, confidence, and self efficiency
7. Resolve subconscious blocks or conflicts
8. To help one remain calm and relaxed while taking examinations

One of the areas which may be a block to learning is some long ago past experience. For example, a child knocks over a glass of milk and is called "stupid." The subconscious mind may accept that as true for the child may take the words literally. The parent may have meant: clumsy, awkward, not paying attention, but used the word, "stupid." If his subconsciously accepts this statement as true, the person will continue to do stupid things. They may have a high IQ, but do poorly in school, because a stupid person cannot make good grades.

Sometimes a teacher will say, "You do good in spelling, but you will never make it in math." The person may develop a problem with math. "Your sister was good in spelling, but you can't spell." The person may develop a spelling problem.

These are some problems that may call for more in depth counseling and hypnotherapy, but most people can improve by proper use of suggestion, imagery, and healing stories.

(1) Randall's Case History

Randall had to have a two point grade average in order to play on his high school basketball team. He said, "The main reason that I go to school is to play basketball. I am the school's leading scorer, so if I fail to make my grades I will also be letting the team down. I can't keep my mind on my studies. I just want to play basketball and go fishing with my buddies." Randall is close to his mother, but not to his father. His father had a heart attack about two years ago and as a result became distant from his son.

In hypnosis, I had Randall imagine the basketball gym door was locked. Whenever he came to play or practice, the door was locked. There was only one key to the gym and that was good grades. Being motivated to study and make good grades is your key to the gym. Your interest in studying is increasing for you want to always have your key to the gym ready to use.

(2) Enjoying School Work

You are ready to enjoy some very pleasant changes in the way you study. Many people have found that if something is boring, tiring, monotonous, or tedious that just a slight change can make that same thing surprisingly pleasant, enjoyable and interesting . . . School work, when completed can give you a sense of accomplishment and doing well, It is your key to the gym door.

When you are just beginning your school work, the feeling is that is going to be done, is being done, and has been done. You have a feeling of expectation that enables you to concentrate better, learn more rapidly and really enjoy studying. Think it over . . . Don't agree yet . . . Think it over before you agree . . . You can actually enjoy doing your assignments and you can feel really proud in knowing that you have completed your school work . . .

There are times when you enjoy being you . . . Being the person in your body . . . Feeling relaxed . . . Feeling comfortable . . . While in your mind you can explore thoughts and ideas that really give you pleasure . . . Now feel a sense of accomplishment, enabling you to go to bed, to sleep peacefully and know your school work is done for the day. Your key to the gym door is safely in your possession.

The image of you completing your school work is a good thing to accomplish . . . And it keeps becoming easier and more enjoyable for you to make good grades . . . The nice feelings come as you are doing it . . . causing it to be really worthwhile. Is that right? I expect your mind to translate everything I'm saying into your own words . . . Your phrases . . . and your own actions . . . so the changes you are accomplishing in your own way . . . not mine . . . You find pleasure in getting your assignments done and in making good grades . . .

Notice that you are already beginning to feel enthusiastic about school . . . You are already sensing that good grades are your key to the gym door. You experience feelings of satisfaction knowing that you are making good grades. You are already organizing the words I have told you into your own actions, and you are pleased to find this continuing after you come out of this hypnotic state.

(3) Improving Memory and Study Habits

You can concentrate on what you are studying. Visualize yourself studying, remembering and recalling what you study. You can make concentration a habit. Your mind is like a computer. You feed data into it by reading and listening. You hear something and record it. You experience something and record it. You can picture the things you read. You can hear the things you see. You can feel the things you hear, you can experience the things you study. Everything fed into your computer is permanently retained and available to you at all times.

You have a good memory and day by day your memory is getting better and better. It is easy for you to learn and remember. Concentration strengthens your mind and memory. Whenever you use your memory, it becomes stronger every time you use it. Every time you study, your concentration and memory enhance your capacity for a successful, creative and productive life.

Whenever you take an exam or when you desire to remember specific information, you are relaxed and calm. Memory comes to the conscious mind much easier when you are relaxed. Therefore, whenever you desire to relax, just close your eyes and take a deep breath. You breathe in relaxation and exhale tension. This relaxes you and enables you to recall the things you have learned.

During an exam, if you come to a question, but do not recall it, just take a deep breath and think, "I know the answer to the question and I am able to recall it in a minute or two." Move on to the next question, and as you work on other questions, the answer comes to the question you had difficulty answering. If you need to go back to a question, you can say, "My mind is like a computer. What I have studied is in the computer. I visualize a computer keyboard and punch the recall button. As I do the answer comes on the screen of my memory."

At the count of three, you come out of the hypnotic state. One. Study, remember, recall, Two. Study, remember, recall. Three.

Chapter Twenty-Three

Pain Management and Enhancing Healing

In using hypnosis to reduce and eliminate pain, it must be remembered that pain is a warning that something is wrong. I use hypnosis to reduce pain and enhance healing when referred to me by the client's physician. I use self hypnosis to relieve pain for myself when I would use an aspirin or some non-prescription medication. If I were to have a recurring pain, such as a headache, I would go to a physician for a check-up.

In a newspaper article, "No Hocus Pocus: Hypnotizing Your Way Out Of Pain," an A.P. writer, writes that for some the word "hypnosis" may conjure images of magic acts. *Mature Outlook* magazine reports that today's version of mind over matter has a more practical spin—helping people control their chronic pain. "Nearly all major centers like to use non-invasive techniques when at all possible," says Dr. Berthold Wolff, a psychologist and director of New York University Comprehensive Pain Center, "Hypnosis is one method whereby the patients can help themselves."

"Basically, hypnosis is a contract between a patient and the doctor (or the therapist to whom the doctor has referred the client). You can never make someone do something against their will." He explains, "We try to teach individuals how to get control. Then it's always easier to deal with the pain."

There are two general classification of pain: acute and chronic. Acute pain is associated with the sudden outset of pain such as a broken arm, a cut finger, a burn on the hand and is generally more intense than chronic pain. Chronic pain is usually of an ongoing nature such as back pain, arthritis, and intensity may vary.

The experience of pain is a combination of the type of pain, tension, fear, and anxiety. Often tension, fear and anxiety can intensify the experience of pain. Pain causes tension and tightening up of the affected area of the body. Our normal response to pain is to resist the pain by tightening up even more and becoming more tense. This increases the severity of the pain experience. By relaxation of the body there is a natural reduction of pain. By proper suggestion in the hypnotic state, the experience of pain can be reduced or eliminated for periods of time. I teach the client self hypnosis and imagery so that client can use it when needed. When working to reduce pain, I do not use the word *pain* for the word itself may increase the symptoms. I use words like "discomfort" or "tension." Hypnosis is very effective in enhancing the healing process or helping the individual better handle a terminal disease.

(1) Devone's Case History

Devone was on the surgery schedule for the next day. Completing my surgery schedule visitations, I came to Devone's room. As I had known Devone for several years, we talked for awhile and I asked him about his surgery, "Is this your fifth or sixth surgery?" "It will be my sixth. You remember that you helped me with hypnosis for pain control after my last surgery?" I nodded "yes" and he continued, "I would really like for you to do that again. I know that you need a doctor's consult so I asked my doctor to put it on my chart." I responded, "Yes," the nurse told me so, "I would like to begin today to prepare you for surgery and again after your surgery."

I explained to him that there was several advantages to pre- and post-operative hypnosis. The advantages are: (1) Reduces pre-operative stress and relaxes the body so you can sleep better tonight. (2) During surgery, fewer chemicals and anesthesia are needed. (3) There tends to be less blood loss during surgery. (4) Patients experience less post-operative nausea and vomiting. (5) The return of normal physiological functions such as urination and bowel movements. (6) Wounds heal more rapidly and patient has a smoother and shorter recovery period.

(2) Pre And Post Operation Suggestion

Tonight, you relax and sleep soundly. You feel relaxed and comfortable in every way for your surgery . . . As you relax peaceful and comfortable, I want to share with you a two step exercise you can do to help go through this surgery successful and heal rapidly. The first step involves focusing on the way your body feels during surgery.

Imagine your body limp and relaxed. The more relaxed you are the better you are prepared for surgery. You know you're being closely observed by skilled doctors and you can safely relax. The anesthesia is administered carefully and safely. The more relaxed you are, the less amount of anesthesia you need for the surgery. This is good for you. The operation is performed skillfully.

Though you are relaxed and unaware consciously during surgery, there is one part of you that remains alert. That part is your body's protector system. That system can keep the wound dry, clean, and free of infection. It can also minimize bleeding, reduce discomfort and promote healing. By letting your body flow along with the surgery with your defense system alert and focused on protection and healing . . . You are working in cooperation with the surgeon to cure your illness.

The second step of the exercise involves focusing on the way your body is to behave after surgery . . . This is for your recovery and convalescence. Prior to surgery, the two steps for the exercise are done together. Once surgery is over, you only concentrate on the second step; the recovery . . .

When you awaken after surgery, you awaken quietly and comfortably as though awakening from a long, peaceful, healthy restoring sleep. When you come out of the anesthesia knowing that surgery is over, once again put yourself in a state of hypnosis. Focus on alerting your defense system to promote healing. Your natural body processes are keeping the wound dry, clean and free of infection. Minimize bleeding and reduce discomfort.

You have prompt and regular bowel movement and prompt and regular urination. You feel pleasantly hungry, vigorous, full of life, pep and vitality. You first awaken in the Recovery Room which is the safest place for you to be. Concentrate on a rapid return to normal functioning, to a stable and comfortable blood pressure. Imagine getting back to a healthy, happy lifestyle as your body heals . . . You feel yourself getting hungry, feeling thirsty, going to the toilet. Think about getting back to a healthy lifestyle as your body heals.

Thus far you've thought about the way your body is to behave during your stay in the hospital. Now I want you to think about the most important behavior. I want you to imagine the things you do, without discomfort or worry, once you've recovered. I want you to imagine yourself doing the things you're eager to do. That's the reason you've come for surgery. You've come to repair a part of your body that is troubling you so you can do the things you want to do, without fear and concern.

For a minute, think about what I've said and then I'll teach you how to bring yourself out of trance so that all of these messages stay with your body. Before I show you how to come out of trance, let's take the time to review your exercise. The first step focusses on the way your body is to behave during surgery; the second, on the way your body is to behave after surgery. Before surgery, you do both steps. After surgery, you do only the second step.

In the first step, you think about the way your body is to behave during surgery. It is to be relaxed and limp, except for the defense system. That system is alert in order to keep the wound dry, clean, and free of infection, and to minimize bleeding and reduce discomfort. Although the anesthesiologist provides whatever amount of anesthesia your body requires, you can make it easier by letting your body know the way to behave; help it flow along with the surgery so you and the surgeon work together to cure your illness.

The second step focuses on recovery. Your defense system is alert to keep the wound dry, clean and free of infection, and to minimize bleeding and reduce discomfort as the healing takes place. Imagine yourself as you regain all normal functioning-your blood pressure rapidly stabilizes and returns to normal. You feel your appetite return. You get thirsty. You sense yourself going to the toilet. You feel eager to move around. Each time before you come out of trance think about the future-the real reason for going through surgery . . . Imagine yourself doing things that you want to do once surgery is over and you have recovered.

As you rest peacefully and calmly, you know God constantly watches over you and you are able to place your trust in His infinite goodness. Now, you are ready to sleep, you sleep soundly and sleep well and wake up sound in body, sound in mind, sound in spirit, and sound in health. You progressively improve, physically, emotionally, and spiritually. Day by day in every way, you are getting better and better, healthier and healthier, stronger and stronger.

When you have finished practicing self-hypnosis, you bring yourself out of trance by saying "at the count of three, come out of this hypnotic state,´progressively improving. One, two, three . . . Now you may come out of hypnosis and either go into a naturally, normal sleep or be wide awake at the count of three. One, healing properly; two, healthier and healthier, three.

The day after surgery, I returned to follow up with post-operative hypnosis.

(3) Reducing Pain Experience

I wonder, as you continue relaxing more and more, if you would enjoy remembering a time when you were completely free from discomfort . . . That was a very enjoyable time for you, and you can enjoy it again if you choose to do so, or you may prefer merely recalling an experience during your childhood when you were at a park or playground having a good time playing on the swing, or playing games with other children . . .

Who knows how much more comfortable you can keep feeling? I don't really know for sure . . . I'm quite certain you feel progressively better than you did when we began this session . . . However, just how much better you feel is as unclear to me as it is to you . . . I would be taking a lot of credit for myself if I told you that you're going to feel really comfortable, relaxed, calm, peaceful and at ease just because I have helped you go into a hypnotic state and your subconscious mind is accepting everything I'm telling you and making it true.

Even though your body is continuing to relax more and more with each breath that you take, whatever relief you feel, either now, or when you awaken and even tomorrow, you realize that your own subconscious mind is doing it because you want it to happen . . . I don't know how your subconscious mind can cause that to happen . . . you may have some idea about it, or you may just find yourself feeling more comfortable and more at ease automatically without knowing how it happened.

While your mind is reviewing what I've said to you, you are realizing that today is today, and you know what day this is. Your expectation is increasing, and in a short time you realize that your experience has been changed in a very pleasant way.

(4) Post-Surgery Suggestions

You are continuing to breathe easily and freely, and are experiencing peace of mind . . . The surgery has been completed . . . you are now safely back in bed and your mind realizes that the surgery has been successful. The processes and activities of your body are now functioning perfectly and are healing your body quickly, comfortable, and completely . . . You are being rejuvenated and restored to perfect health . . . Your strength, energy, and vitality continues increasing as your body is healing, and you are pleased with the improvement you experience . . . You are recovering, you experience very pleasant sensations of healing . . . All parts of your body are functioning properly to enable you to heal rapidly and perfectly . . . You are looking forward to total recovery, and you notice improvement in all areas of your life; Physically, mentally and emotionally . . .

Your subconscious mind is causing you to desire foods that provide proper nourishment, strength, energy and vitality to every part of your body where it is needed . . . When you come out of the hypnotic state, you remain calm and relaxed . . . You continue breathing easily and freely . . . You find it easy to continue feeling calm and comfortable . . . Your body processes are carrying just the right amount of blood to the areas where the surgery was performed, and is supplying that area of your body with everything it needs to achieve health . . . As you heal properly, your digestive system functions easily and properly . . . Your bladder and bowels are functioning easily and normally. Fluids pass through your bladder easily . . . All parts of your body are functioning smoothly and perfectly . . . And you continue achieving a rapid and complete recovery. Comfortable, peaceful, healing, day to day in every way you are getting better and better, healthier and healthier, stronger and stronger.

A few days after his release from the hospital, Devone wrote the President of Methodist Hospital. He wrote, "Chaplain Durbin helped me prepare for surgery using hypnosis. He also helped me with pain control following surgery. I have had six surgeries and I had less complications, less pain medication, and healed much faster than ever before."

(5) Mr. Thibodeaux's Case History

Mr. Thibodeaux was a 69-year-old retired electrician who had suffered a stroke. When I first began to work with Mr. Thibodeaux, he could not talk nor move his right arm or leg. A physical therapist suggested to Mr. Thibodeaux's physician that I be consulted to work with Mr. Thibodeaux using hypnosis. After talking with Mr. Thibodeaux about hypnosis, we began therapy.

(6) Stroke Improvement #1: "Rewiring The House"

Allow yourself to drift into a deeper state of relaxation, similar to a dreaming state. While you continue to relax, you can pretend . . . You can pretend you are having a dream . . . You dream that you are an electrician and you have the job of rewiring this house . . . Imagine the house now . . . See the way it looks . . . This house is not completely without power . . . Someone lives there, but some parts of the house is without electricity . . . Some areas of the house wiring needs to be repaired . . . It is your job to go into the house and make all the repairs needed for the house to work properly . . .

You are very skilled at your job . You have all the right equipment and tools needed to complete this job. You have everything you need to make this house work properly . . . Pretend you are walking into the house. First you go into each room and find out how may outlets, lights and switches are there . . . Take as much time as you need in the next 30 seconds of clock time . . .

Now you find out what kind of service is already there . . . Carefully inspecting the breakers and circuits . . . Knowing that each one is important and has a special purpose. Now you decide if the house needs any special lines . . . These lines may not have been there before . . . You may need new lines . . . Take your time and look very closely . . . Now you look at the wiring in the house . . . Decide which wiring is old and needs to be replaced . . . Check the connections on the wiring you decide is OK . . .

You know that the house has some power because some of the lights and outlets are working just fine. You check the breaker that goes to the meter. Make sure it is safe for you to work on this house . . . Now imagine you are making all the necessary repairs and in your imagination you are re-routing certain wires, tying into other lines, making changes as needed to get electricity to all parts of the house . . . Take as much time as you need in the next minute of clock time to complete the rewiring.

You have rewired the house . . . Everything is completed . . . All connections, switches, and lines are in working order . . . Walk through the house, turn on lights . . . Plug in useful appliances . . . Check every detail and enjoy your success. Feel the pride of accomplishment . . . Know that you have rewired the house properly and the lights and outlets are functioning as they should. Enjoying this accomplishment, you gently move into a deeper state of hypnosis . . .

One of the most inspiring statements of Jesus in the entire New Testament are the words, *the Kingdom of God is within you.* Just think for a moment of the tremendous meaning contained in those words . . . Those words mean there is a power within you that can keep you strong at all times. They mean there is a source of wisdom within you that can provide you with guidance in every situation of your life . . . They also mean that you have within you the transforming power of love . . . That your life can be enhanced by letting love flow through you . . .

Your mind can be compared to a house . . . Repairs can be made to any part so that it can work properly . . . And your subconscious mind can understand things you do not consciously understand . . . As you rewired your imaginary house, you can also rewire your brain so that it functions properly . . . The Associated Press reported that scientists have discovered a dramatic reorganization in the human brain that apparently helps some stroke patients overcome paralysis . . .

The study of stroke patients who recovered from paralysis found that impaired portions of their brain had started showing control over movement which was otherwise considered the work of the damaged side of the brain. The study showed, "The human brain is capable of a lot of reorganization following injury, and that is the way in which recovery is established." It is a fact that when one area of the brain has been damaged, even badly damage, that some other related areas of the brain can help take over some of the functions normally coming from the damaged area. This allows the brain to bypass the damaged area, which has acted like a broken electrical wire and rewire around the damaged area to the other side of the brain . . . As in your imagination you rewired the house. You let your subconscious mind rewire your brain to bypass the damaged area so your body can function properly . . .

Your subconscious mind is very powerful . . . It knew just what to do to cause your body to develop . . . To cause you to grow arms and legs . . . To make you male or female and develop all the organs in your body . . . To develop your face and all your sensory organs . . . It even caused you to develop a brain . . . From a single cell . . . It is now finding a way to bring healing and strength to your body and this is a progressive experience as day by day in every way, you are getting better and better, healthier and healthier, stronger and stronger . . .

All of these suggestions are now in the storehouse of your mind . . . They continue working even after you come out of this hypnotic state . . . They continue to be just as powerful and just as strong as you live your daily life . . . Your mind continues to cause your natural healing energies to flow through your body . . . Day by day, your health continues to improve . . .

When I came for the second session, Mr. Thibodeaux moved his right hand and smiled but still no speech.

(7) Stroke Improvement #2: "For Left Brain Damage"

You know that you have been able to perform many functions throughout your life; things like walking and talking and writing and feeding yourself. These became second nature to you many, many years ago. Then, you had this stroke, you found that very suddenly you were unable to do those very things that you have done automatically for decades.

For some time, it has been very confusing and difficult, because of this strange and frustrating situation. In particular, you have had a hard time speaking, because you seem to lose the words that you are looking for. This has been all the more exasperating and depressing because you have been able to talk for so many years.

Your doctor has explained that the stroke affected the left side of your brain, the side where the speech center is located. That is why you are having trouble with your words. However, the right side of your brain is fine. Here is an interesting challenge for you, you can now teach the right side of your brain to do what the left side used to do. This is all the more interesting because the right side of your brain seems to be more active in the realm of imagery, music, and creativity. We know that both sides of the brain can perform all the various functions, and there is a tremendous cross-over in activity.

But this is just what you need. Think of the possibilities! The right side of the brain has all the potential that it needs to learn the various function of the left side of the brain and it has great power and creativity to find a way to resort your speech and activities in the affected arm, hand, and leg. So ask your subconscious mind and your body to get into strong communication in order to cooperated and collaborate fully for your healing. Allow the function of your left brain to be taken over by your right brain.

Did you know that you have a bridge from one side of your brain to the other? It is a strong bridge connecting the two hemispheres of your brain. How wonderful that you have a bridge already there. It can be one of the routes that information can take as it is transferred from the left side to the right.

In your own way, create the image of this bridge in your mind, and visualize or feel or imagine that information is traveling past the blockade and across the bridge, from the left side to the right . . . When it gets to the right side, let it find the exact place to settle; somewhere accessible, where other information coming in can find it easy to move from the left side to the right.

Then, when the information is safely lodged in the right side of the brain, again invoke that wonderful mind/body communication as you direct your right brain to begin to use that information. You can be very, very curious about how that is happening . . . Will you feel like one finger is moving or will it be two or three or even the entire hand? Will it be a few words or entire sentences? Will it happen all at once or will you progressively improve until you are healed and strong . . . Just let it happen . . . (This is an illustration of the use of "will" but the suggestion is not to use "will" remains in effect in most cases.)

We know that this may probably take a very concerned effort over some period of time . . . After all it took you some period of time to learn how to speak, use your arm, hand, and leg in the first place . . . So it is reasonable that it may take some time for your right brain to learn to do what your left brain had been doing . . . Stay patient and calm and let the left side of your brain teach the right side what to do . . .

Remember, too, that there are other ways of transferring information besides sending it across the bridge. Send that information on a passing hormone, for instance. There is great hormone involvement in any learning process. This is another opportunity for mind/body communication and collaboration . . .

And then it may be possible that only the deepest part of your subconscious mind knows about or has access to—so remember to ask your subconscious to use all the information that it has to help you in this project. Progressively you experience improvement, strength, healing, as your left brain activities crosses the bridge to the right side which takes over to bring healing . . .

By the time Mr. Thibodeaux was released from the hospital, he was able to carry on a conversation. He would sometimes be a little hesitant but was talking. He also was walking with a walker and using his hand rather effectively.

(8) Arthur's Case History

Arthur, a 39-year-old business man, came to me following a hospital stay. He had cancer and wanted to use hypnosis and imagery to improve his chances for recovery. He had read an article in a national magazine about the use of hypnosis for enhancing healing and he wanted to use these techniques along with his chemotherapy. He was involved in a regular exercise routine and was taking a variety of vitamins.

Arthur was active in his church and several professional and civic organizations. We discussed the importance of hopeful expectation which he had demonstrated by coming to therapy. I asked him to prepare a list of stressful experiences that he had experienced from six to eighteen months before he knew that he had cancer. After normal pre-talk, we had our first hypnotic session.

After the induction, I had him imagine coming into the hospital for his chemotherapy. He was to imagine that he was looking forward to seeing his nurses and friends at the hospital. He was to realize that each treatment was one less that he had to take. If at any time, he experienced discomfort in his stomach, he could close his eyes and imagine that the fluids in his stomach were red in color and that his natural healing chemicals were going to work to change the red color to clear with comfort coming with the change in color. As the red fades and the stomach fluids become clear, he feels better and better . . . This was for him a very effective way of reducing any stomach discomfort.

(9) Healing Within (adapted from Louis Bauer)

David wrote in the Psalms 46:11, "Be still and know that I am God." That is what you are doing now..Your are learning to be still . . . Allowing your body and your conscious mind to relax through hypnosis enables you to tap into the powerful resources of your subconscious mind . . .

As you continue relaxing now, you can feel that relaxation spreading throughout your entire body. You can feel total relaxation from the top of your head to the bottom of your feet . . . It is like a soft gentle soothing, protective light . . . Gently surrounding you . . . Protecting you . . . Comforting you . . . And with that gentle loving light comes peace . . . That light is coming from God to bring healing to your body and activating your own healing chemicals to work for you . . . Jesus said, *The Kingdom of God is within you.* You have within you the answer to all the questions . . . The solution to all the problems . . . And the healing energies within you to help heal many kinds of illness, sickness or disease . . .

As you continue relaxing now, your mind is at peace and is open to the awareness of the inflow and outflow of God's love . . . You are in the process of making some very important changes that bring you greater happiness, joy, and inner peace . . . You are pleased with the progressive improvement in all areas of your life.

You keep your thoughts positive and you find that attracts happy, healthy conditions to you . . . You meet every challenge in your life with confidence, sureness, and power. Miracles come quietly into the mind that can be still . . . Healing—mental, physical, emotional, and spiritual comes from within . . . You accept guidance from within . . . God is guiding you.

Sit quietly with your eyes closed . . . God's light within you is sufficient . . . It has the power to heal . . . The shining light within you brings peace of mind and hopeful expectation.

In each of us is a spark of the divine . . . God's love is shining its light throughout your body . . . You keep developing a greater attitude of love and understanding . . . Your spiritual awareness is increasing . . . Your self-confidence, self-acceptance, self-esteem, and self-awareness keep increasing more and more each day . . . You notice improvements—mentally, emotionally, physically, and spiritually . . . Just be still . . .

Your mind can sort out all of those secrets, feelings, imprints, impressions, thoughts and ideas, including those you are not consciously aware of . . . Your subconscious mind can examine them and in its own way work out a very pleasant solution for you..It is a nice thing to learn, because it enables you to do the things you need to do..So continue relaxing peacefully and calmly . . .

You are a very special, very unique, one of a kind person. God made you: body, mind, and spirit; and He made you in His image . . . You are being strengthened and rejuvenated by the Divine healing power of love . . .

(10) Protective Ants (adapted from Havens and Walters)

There is a tree in Africa that has a special relationship with a particular kind of ant. The ants spend their entire lives living on that tree. They build their nests out of its leaves, they only drink the particular kind of sap that tree produces and secretes and eat the special tiny berries it grows. They never leave that tree because that tree provides everything they need.

And this type of ant is the only insect that does live on that tree. Whenever any other insect begins to crawl upon it or lands on one of its leaves, the ant sentries send out an alarm and all the other ants come running. They attack those foreign bodies and either destroy them or drive them away and, in this way they protect that tree from any invaders that might attack it or even destroy them or drive them away and in this way they protect the tree from invaders that might attack it or destroy it. They save the tree and the tree saves them.

We have within our bodies an immune system that functions much like the ants who take care of that tree, automatically and continuously, rushing to do those things needed to heal and protect.

As the ants protects the tree, your body's immunity and healing capabilities are working rapidly to bring healing to your body. This is already working in your body, because you want it to work . . . and your subconscious mind is cooperating with your conscious desire to be healthy and strong. Your entire organism is responding and your health continues to improve.

And all of those processes function by receiving directions from your subconscious mind . . . Thus, the more positive your subconscious mind is programmed, the healthier your body becomes . . . That's one of the reasons it is so important for you to develop a positive, loving attitude about yourself . . .

So each day your self-confidence, your self-acceptance, and your self-esteem keeps increasing, and you continue realizing more and more of your own self-worth.

William James the psychologist wrote, "The greatest discovery of my generation is that human beings, by changing the inner attitudes of their minds, can change the outer aspects of their lives." Bernie S. Siegal said, "My own day-to-day clinical experience has convinced me that the state of mind changes the state of the body by working through the central nervous system, the endocrine system and the immune system . . . Peace of mind sends the body a live message. Thus, all healing is scientific, even though science can't yet explain exactly how the unexpected occurs."

That is backed up by a statement in the Bible that says, *You can be transformed by the renewing of your mind.* By properly using your mind, you can have a good effect on your health. Now just allow your subconscious mind to cause you to relax more peacefully and calmly. As you relax, you allow your body to keep improving physically. The organs, glands and normal functions of the body begin to work properly. As you feel better about yourself, you eat the foods that are right for your body. You eat foods that cause your body to be healthy and strong. You exercise according to what your doctor suggests for you. Exercise helps you reduce the effect of stress on your body and improves your health.

As you relax, your subconscious mind is giving direction to each cell of your body to function in unison and harmony with other cells to eliminate harmful cells by your natural body processes to bring healing to your body. Imagine and visualize your body healthy. The wise old man of Proverbs said, *"Whatsoever a person thinks in his/her heart, so is he/she."* The images you hold in your mind you tend to become. As you relax and use your imagination, you increase your natural body healing chemicals and endorphins which bring healing and comfort to your body. You are learning to use your mind and imagination along with proper medical care to bring healing to your body.

At the next session, Arthur has a list of stressful events that had taken place in his life as I had requested: (1) Father died eight months before he was diagnosed with cancer, (2) Rigors of his business life, (3) He was in the fifth year of a lawsuit against him, (4) I tend to hold my emotions in and that ties me up inside, and (5) I don't have enough time for my family. We discussed each of these areas to include how to handle these for his benefit.

For the next session, I asked him to bring in a list of benefits he received from his illness. When I asked him for the list, he said, "I don't get any benefits so I don't have a list." I asked him to think about this for awhile because one generally gets some benefits or secondary gains from their illnesses. I pointed out to him that this was not being done to make him feel guilty, but to let him see that he can play apart in his health by this attitudes and actions.

For benefits Arthur wrote: (1) Has enough money to live comfortably without working, (2) Doesn't have to put up with the pressure of business, and (3) More time with family. We discussed how he could reap these benefits without being sick. Over the next four weeks, I used a number of scripts in working with Arthur. Among them are the following (I closed with "Love, Joy, and Hope").

(11) Hypnotic Suggestions for Overcoming Cancer

Allow yourself to become very warm and comfortable. Let any fear fade away . . . becoming very warm and relaxed . . . safe and secure. Begin your healing journey by first making yourself very small, as small as a drop of water, and then slip inside a clear bubble that protects you and supply you with everything you need. Allow yourself to become even smaller now and enter your bloodstream.

Circulate through your body and tell your immune system to release stronger and more effective white blood cells into your bloodstream. Let these white blood cells be represented by an animated or symbolic form. Watch them swim through your bloodstream, full of energy and sure of their purpose . . . to dissolve any unhealthy growth that they find. If you would like you can transmit messages of encouragement or directions to your immune system. You might want to thank your immune system for the good job it is doing in the face of a challenger . . . or ask your immune system if there is anything you can do to help speed your healing.

You have a strong ally in your chemotherapy helping you fight any diseased cells. Your chemotherapy and your own immune system are stronger than any diseased cells and your system is destroying the diseased cells. The defeated diseased cells are being released from your body by your natural elimination system. Imagine that you are being completely healed and then watch your immune system cells patrol through your body in a loving and protective way. Imagine and feel yourself being restored to a state of good health and appreciate and love yourself for taking the time to heal in this way . . .

(12) Healing Imagery

God has created in all living things the most incredible ability to heal . . . Think of the many times in your life when a wound, an illness, an injury has healed for you. You have a marvelous healing energy within you . . .

Go now, deep within yourself: the very center of yourself, which God created in you, to the source of that healing energy within you. Go to the very source of that healing energy, be aware of that energy that comes from the very center of yourself. Gather up that energy, and direct it to that part of your body where you instinctively know it must be directed!

Each one of us has his or her own personal concept of that healing energy. For me, it is God's healing light, like the sun, a light that can be directed to the part of the body which needs healing, and cover that part of the body with its healing glow. It is a golden light, that surrounds and bathes the ill or wounded part of the body with that healing golden energy.

Discover your own concept of what your healing energy is. Locate it deep within you, and direct it to wherever your body needs it. Now FEEL, SENSE that healing that is already beginning within you. You can actually experience and feel that healing. That's right. Direct that energy through your body, to wherever you intuitively know it is needed . . . Knowing that you may even be surprised at the part of your body which you have intuitively chosen! You are aware that the subconscious mind has so much more information than the conscious mind has. The subconscious mind may know that some other part of the body, different from where your conscious mind would have thought, may need that healing first. Trust your subconscious mind to direct that energy; trust your response.

Now let your wonderful, creative imagination formulate an image, in your awareness, of what that ill or wounded part of your body is like . . . what it looks like, or feels like, or indeed even sounds like . . .

Then place that image, in your inner awareness, on one side. Now, begin to create another image: This image is of healing, of convalescence, or recovery. It is the image of what your body is like when you are healed, feels like, sounds like when you are well again; restore harmony and power to your body. Fill in all of that wonderful imagery with detail, in whatever kind of image is right for you, remembering that the image can be realistic or symbolic, two-or three dimensional, whatever you instinctively know is connected with your deep sense of self.

Now let the image of healing and health take over completely. The healing image is completely wiping out the old image and that is what you picture in your mind from now on . . . The healing images is victorious. Picture in your mind from now on . . . The healing image is victorious. Picture yourself as well and doing all the things you want to do.

In your own self hypnosis every day, reinforce this healing imagery. Keep the healthy image in your mind . . . The more frequently you do that, the stronger the message that you are giving your subconscious mind and hence your body . . . Say to yourself now and many times each day, both in and out of the hypnotic state, "Day by day in every way, I am getting better and better, healthier and healthier, and happier and happier."

(13) Love, Joy, and Hope

Let the music fill you with a sense of tranquility. Let it carry you gently to your special place where you can use all of your senses; visual, auditory, and feelings, to make the imagery more powerful to you . . . So now let's take a moment, a moment that you're entitled to . . . and start on a journey to those places where you feel like celebrating. Let love, joy, and hope enter your life . . . Take a moment . . . to breath in love . . . breath in joy . . . breath in hope . . . Love, joy and hope are real . . . They are all available to you . . . Notice what these qualities do to your body . . . and your mind . . . as you breath them in . . . And when you breath out, let go . . . Let the tension go . . . Relax the jaw muscles . . . Rest your eyelids and just keep them closed . . . Let the back and neck muscles relax . . . They carry a burden . . . But let the back and neck muscles relax . . . They carry a burden but let the burden roll off your shoulders . . . Breathe in relaxation and exhale tension and let relaxation and love move down through your body . . . Be aware of it . . . love it . . . and relax it . . .

Be aware of love . . . You are learning to love yourself. You like yourself . . . You are realizing that loving yourself is not selfish. Selfishness is the opposite of self-love. A selfish person does not love himself and lacks self-worth.

A perfect example of this lack of self-worth and selfishness in seen in the popular character of J.R. Ewing of the old TV show "Dallas." The only way J. R. could feel good about himself was to put someone down . . . to beat the other person in business deal, or to get another person into trouble. Poor J. R. didn't love himself, therefore, he was unable to love others.

As you begin to love yourself, you see your worth as a person and you can better relate to and love others. Perhaps that is what Jesus meant by *"Love your neighbor as yourself."* As you love yourself, you can conquer destructive forces of negative thinking, worry, resentment, fear, and anxiety. Let love, joy and hope fill your life . . . Just feel the peace filling your life and body . . . And how good that feels . . . Just relax . . . Just allow the relaxation to move through your body . . . Relaxing the muscles . . . relieving discomfort . . . Give an extra measure of love to very part of your body that is having difficulty of one kind or another . . . You can love yourself . . . Just love yourself . . . until you are filled with love . . . Make sure that every cell is open to love . . . And see any problems being breathed out or eliminated in anyway that is comfortable for you . . . And take a moment to purify and cleanse your body and mind in a way that feels right to you . . .

Let joy be experienced within you . . . At the very center of your being. David wrote in Psalm 30, "O Lord, you have turned my lament into dancing, you have stripped off my sack cloth and clothed me with joy." In Psalm 149, David continues, "Let the children of Zion be joyful in their king. Let them praise his name in dance, let them sing praises unto him with the tumbrel and harp." With joyful dancing and singing, David closes his Psalms, "Praise ye the Lord. Praise God in his sanctuary, praise him in the firmament of his power, Praise him for his mighty acts, praise him according to his excellent greatness, praise him with the sound of the trumpet, praise him with Psaltery and harp, praise him with the tumbrel and dance . . . Let everything that hath breath praise the Lord, Praise ye the Lord." Feel total love . . . Total acceptance . . . Total joy . . . Total hope . . .

Take as much time as you need in the next one minute of clock time to explore the many things you have to be joyful about. As you do so mentally dance the dance of joy. The Snoopy of Peanuts is often leaping and dancing for joy. On one occasion Snoopy begins to dance about and shout, "To dance is to live." and then, "I feel sorry for people who cannot dance." In the last frame, he goes on dancing joyfully and says, "If you can't dance, at least be able to do a happy hop." I would like to add one frame to that cartoon, "If you can't dance with your feet, at least be able to dance in your heart." This is a picture of wholesome living.

St. Paul wrote to the Hebrews, "Faith is the assurance of things hoped for, the evidence of things not seen." In Romans, Paul wrote, "Let hope keep you joyful; in trouble stand firm, persist in prayer." Paul is suggesting that you live your life in hopeful expectation of what is not yet but can be.

Hope it the outreach of our inner life for courage, meaning, and wholeness. Hope is the reality which transforms mere existence or even self-destructive tendencies to a life lived by positive affirmation. This positive life affirmation is more than just giving lip service to hope but it is a way of life. Sometimes our hoping is for something specific while at others times, it is more our oneness to life's opportunities. As you hope, you live in a world of open doors and hopeful expectation for the good life.

Live in hope for in so doing you tap into spiritual forces which can help you meet this situation to either overcome or endure. Someone once said, "If you can imagine it, you can possess it. If you can dream it, you can become it. If you can envision it, you can attain it. If you can picture it, you can achieve it." It is yours as you imagine, dream, envision, and picture it.

Now continue to relax and enjoy who you are . . . Love yourself, live in joy, experience hope . . . . Live in love, live in joy, live in hope for you have gotten this far . . . You have survived . . . You have made it and you now have more love, more joy, and more hope in your life . . . You choose to celebrate life, love, joy, and hope . . . Know that whatever questions may come to you that love is the answer . . . experience, love, joy, and hope as you come out of this hypnotic state . . .

(14) Dr. Hodges' Tongue Bite

An interesting incident occurred at a recent seminar sponsored by the Health and Welfare Board of the Louisiana Conference of the United Methodist Church. During the lunch break, Dr. Richard Hodges, Director of Methodist Children's Home of New Orleans, bit his tongue. As the seminar was held at Pendleton Memorial Methodist Hospital, I was taking the break in my office. Richard came into my office and said, "Paul, I bit my tongue and it will not stop bleeding." He was holding a paper towel to his mouth. On his tongue was an area about the size of my small finger nail and it was bleeding like a gusher.

I asked him to set down in my recliner. I used an eye fixation induction and gave suggestion that the bleeding would stop and quick, effective healing would begin. The blood going to the area of the bite would be diverted to other parts of the tongue and healing occurs rapidly and quickly. I counted him out of hypnosis and asked him to open his mouth. There was no blood to be seen and I could barely tell where the bite had been. All I could say to him was to go to the men's room across the hall from my office and look at his tongue. He said, "Well it doesn't hurt anymore." He got up for the chair and went across the hall to the men's room. He looked at this tongue's reflection in the mirror and said, "This is astonishing." As he had purchased a copy of my book, *Human Trinity Hypnotherapy,* a few months before, he continued, "I am going to read your book again. This is astonishing." At the beginning of the afternoon session of the seminar, he shared the incident with those in attendance. The entire hypnotic session lasted less than three minutes. (Dr. Hodges gave me permission to use his real name in reporting this story.)

CHAPTER TWENTY-FOUR
AGE REGRESSION

When using age regression, I suggest to the client, you always hear and understand me no matter where you are or what your age. You always see me being a very close and dear friend who you can confide in easily and comfortable. You always communicate with me in a manner that you know I can understand. Is that all right with you? If it is alright with the client I proceed. Closely associate with finding the cause of a problem is generally a three fold search. For this I use the Hypnoanalysis model.

1. The Initial Sensitizing Event is not recallable by the conscious mind.
    a. The individual is sensitized by an emotionally powerful past incident but no symptom appears
    b. Not always easy to find and not always necessary to find, but individual may be subject to reoccurrence of symptoms if not dealt with and released
2. The Symptom Producing Event is when symptoms begin to appear and may or may not be recalled.
    a. A second emotionally powerful event that trigger symptom
    b. Not always apparently related to the first
3. The Symptom Intensifying Event is an intensifying of symptoms.
    a. Recallable
    b. May or may not be different from previous experiences
    c. Often causes the person to seek help

When using age regression be aware that if the client experiences emotional trauma, the client may experience an abreaction. If the client begins to cry, move about, shows fear, stick with them, remain calm, and either allow the client to work through it or help her move away from the situation. This can be done by having them see it as if on TV and suggestions for reducing the emotional impact. An abreaction may lead to healing and the release of tension.

(1) False Memories

Another point of caution. When one relives a past event the memory may or may not be accurate fact. Memories can be fabricated either by the therapist or the client. At a meeting of the American Psychological Association, Elizabeth Lobtus, an authority on memory stated, "The idea of repression of early traumatic memories is a concept many psychotherapist readily accept." She goes on to say that there is evidence to suggest that the "Memories" are false ones, implanted by therapists through the power of suggestion and then uncritically accepted by them as evidence of truth.

She blamed the theory of the book, *The Courage to Heal* which suggest the abuse probably occurred even if the person has no memory of it and that any demands of corroboration are not reasonable. Loftus stated that her research indicates that it is easy to implant false memories. she said, "That so many individuals enter therapy with no memory of abuse but accepts memories during therapy naturally makes one wonder about what might be happening in therapy."

A woman came to me stating that she has been to a psychiatrist who regressed her back to a supposed sexual molestation by her father. She was considering confronting her father and accusing him of sexual abuse when she was a little girl. Before doing that, she wanted a second opinion because in the conscious state, she has no memory of the abuse . . . She had always felt very close to her father and was never consciously afraid of him.

In a regression, I asked her to go back to any experience from the past that can clarify her situation in relation to her father. She want back to a situation that occurred when she was a three-year-old and continued for about two years. She used to like to have her dad rock her on his foot which she called, "riding the horsey." During this time of play, she experienced sexual pleasure and orgasms. Of the first experience, she said, "Daddy is holding my hands while I ride the horsey and it feels good between my legs. Something is happening, if feels so good, but I don't understand. The good feeling is coming from where I pee pee from." I asked her, "Is there anyone else in the room with you and your father?" She replied, "Yes, my mama and my brother." From these regressions, it appears that her father was totally innocent of any abuse and was just playing a normal child game with his daughter the same way he had played with her older brother who wanted to "ride the horsey."

She was satisfied that her father had not abused her in anyway and was indeed just having a good time with his daughter without being aware of her experiencing any sexual feeling. As a therapist be sure that you do not put ideas or contribute to false memories. The reliving of false memories has destroyed many good men and women.

(2) Bill's Case History

Bill came to see me because he was having trouble developing a meaningful relationship with a person of the opposite sex. Bill also confessed that he was a workaholic and this had been a leading cause of the break up of his first marriage. I worked with Bill for several weeks for stress management and self-confidence.

(3) Self-confidence and Relationship Improvement

As you continue relaxing more, it is not important for you to consciously listen to my words . . . In fact, you don't even need to consciously pay any attention to what I'm saying because the subconscious levels of your mind can hear everything I say, and enable you to respond automatically, without any conscious effort by you.

Even though it is a fact that you have the power and the ability to achieve any goal you want to achieve, there are certain actions you can take that enable you to progress more rapidly and without interfering with your relationships. One of the most important actions you can take is already happening . . . You find that permitting yourself to be hypnotized is one of the most helpful, most beneficial actions you can take for increasing your self-confidence, and helping you in all other areas of your life . . . How you feel about yourself is reflected in how you relate to others. You are learning to love yourself and thereby you are more loving and thoughtful toward others . . .

In the past, you may have had doubts about your abilities to accomplish things without over working yourself and thereby failing to place proper priorities . . . But now that your confidence is increasing rapidly, you have the confidence you need for every situation or circumstances that come up in your life . . .

You find your confidence increasing each day . . . You believe in yourself as being a person who possesses the knowledge, the wisdom, and the ability to achieve the goals you want to achieve . . . and at the same time be responsive to your loved ones and friends . . . In the past you may have had doubts, but those doubts are rapidly fading away . . . All doubts are soon gone completely, . . . Those doubts are being released and are being replaced with a strong sense of confidence . . . You are beginning to realize your own self-worth . . . You are a very special person . . . You have special talents and capabilities to meet your needs . . . Each day you are continuing to develop a greater realization of your capabilities . . . You are progressing rapidly by using a technique that keeps reinforcing and strengthening your concept of yourself . . . And it keeps increasing your self-confidence, your self-acceptance and self-reliance . . .

You have outstanding capabilities . . . You possess a tremendous power that you can use to be a success . . . Each day your determination to use the power of your mind to help you attain greater success and better your relationship with women keeps increasing . . . Repeat that idea silently in your mind now . . . "Each day I use the power of my mind to help me attain greater understanding of women and how to relate to women so that meaningful relationships can develop . . . "

You can do anything you make up your mind to do . . . By using the power of your mind in a positive way, you draw to yourself everything that benefits you in a helpful way including relating to women in a positive caring way . . . Think these words in your mind now, "I believe in myself . . . I believe I can achieve what I desire into reality . . ." You find it beneficial to keep repeating those statements over to yourself several times each day, especially just before going to sleep and just after you wake up . . . Your self-confidence continues increasing more each day . . . And you recognize that you are attracting the attention of people who recognize you as a capable, loving person . . .

You are aware that you attract to you what you think and believe, so you keep your thoughts on goals you want to achieve and other positive ideas that are beneficial to you and bring you greater happiness, and enjoyment, and prosperity . . .

One of the most important goals in life is to keep becoming a better person, you can do that by being the positive self-confident, self-assured person you are capable of being . . . Self confidence and proper concern for others increases your abilities to establish and maintain meaningful relationships . . . You can do it . . . Walter D. Wintle wrote a poem which I would like to read the last stanza to you,

"Life's battles don't always go
to the stronger or faster man (woman)
But sooner or later the man (woman) who wins
Is the fellow (lady) who thinks he (she) can."

You have outstanding capabilities . . . You have within you tremendous mental and creative powers to succeed and develop good lasting relationship . . . So your motivation is increasing . . . Your confidence is increasing . . . and you have the courage you need to achieve more and more happiness, love and joy in your life . . .

(4) Bill's Age Regression

During one of our sessions, we did an age regression. I asked Bill to go back to the cause of his problem. He went back to a situation when he was seven years old. His father was dying of cancer and he told young Bill that he would have to be a big boy and take care of his mother. This was the Initial Sensitizing Event (ISE).

The second event that he went to in the regression was a time in high school when he had to choose between a job and playing baseball at his high school. Due to the family situation, he chose to work instead of playing baseball. This was the Symptom Producing Event (SPE).

As a result of being a compulsive worker as an adult, he spent so much time on his job that he neglected his wife. Even though she told him time and time again that she wanted more of his time, he would not change. Finally, she divorced him because of his lack of attention. This was the Symptom Intensifying Event (SIE). Over the next few sessions, I had him go back in his imagination and nurture the "little boy" of his past and releasing the "little boy" within from the damaging effect of his father's statement, "You are going to have to be a big boy and take care of your mother."

After we worked on releasing other things that contributed to his workaholic, I told him the story of the Stairway to Nowhere.

(5) Stairway to Nowhere

I would like to share with you a story by Thomas Witherspoon about a man who built for himself the finest house in the neighborhood. He spared no expense in planning, purchasing material and for construction of the house. He was an unusual man and some might call him eccentric. His unusual imagination revealed itself in one very strange feature in his house, which was a stairway in the living room. Now, if you have a second floor, or even an attic, a stairway would not be so unusual, but this house had no second floor or attic. The stairway simply went to the ceiling and stopped right there.

For most of those who saw it, the stairway served no useful purpose at all, but to the homeowner, it was a thing of beauty. Although others may question his sanity for building a stairway to nowhere, he was very serious about it. Another individual who was very concerned about the stairway was the local building inspector. When he examined the house and before he gave it official sanction for dwelling purposes, he asked the owner, "Why a stairway and where does it go?" The owner replied, "I simply wanted a stairway and it doesn't go anywhere." The building inspector quickly responded, "Well, before I can approve your home, you're going to have to put a bannister on the stairway. It's a safety hazard without one." The owner complied and a bannister was added.

That stairway to nowhere might sound foolish, but the owner of that house is not the only person to build a stairway to nowhere. Many of us build stairways to nowhere by expending our energy in areas that are harmful to us or by limiting our lives. You have the opportunity today to get off your stairway to nowhere. You can begin today to live a successful life and to enjoy the life you have. You can be accepted as you are without having to work so hard to be accepted.

Bill last came to me for a session in 1987. Since then he has married and is enjoying a happy marriage. He makes a good living financially, but he now spends time with his wife and two stepdaughters, so he is enjoying his living. I closed his last session with "New ways of seeing yourself" and "Eagle and Chickens with two endings."

(6) New Ways of Seeing Yourself

Sometime in the past, you accepted a statement by someone about your abilities. You accepted that verdict as true and you have lived your life based upon that statement. Now, you can look at that situation from a different vantage point and that can provide you with an opportunity to change.

Dr. A. Dudly Dennison tells a story about Dr. A.J. Cronin and how he overcame his feelings of inferiority which he had been living with for years. When Cronin was in medical school, one of his professors told him that his performance in surgery was unacceptable. The professor told him that he might become a general physician, but never a surgeon. At that moment, Cronin accepted his professors's judgement and from that time on focused on the general practice of medicine. When he finished his medical training, he went to a remote areas of the Scottish Highlands. He was the only physician within a hundred miles.

During a storm, a large tree fell on the son of the local pastor crushing his spine. Dr. Cronin was afraid to do the necessary surgery. The words of his old professor that he would never make a surgeon were ringing in his ears. The boy's father begged him to operate for without surgery, his son would be permanently paralyzed. Cronin said, "For the first time, I questioned the validity of the professor's verdict. Doubts and fears were swept away. I knew I could operate successfully and with God's help, I did."

From that experience, Dr. Cronin was able to change his mind about himself that he could not do surgery which was based upon his professor's statement. You can also change. You do not have to continue living with that false belief that you have to always be working. You can have time for a relationship. Your subconscious mind is assisting you by working out a very pleasant solution for you. As you accept a new understanding of your self-worth, you continue to make happy and healthy changes in your life and it is so.

(7) Eagle and Chicken with Two Endings (Which Will You Choose?)

A man found an eagle's egg and put it in a nest of a barnyard hen. The eaglet hatched with the brood of chicks and grew up with them. All his life, the eagle did what the barnyard chickens did, thinking he was a barnyard chicken. He scratched the earth for worms and insects. He clucked, cackled, and would thrash his wings and fly a few feet into the air. Years passed and the eagle grew to adulthood. One day he saw a magnificent bird high above him in a cloudless sky. It glided in graceful majesty among the powerful wind currents with scarcely beat of its strong golden wings.

(First Ending)

The eagle looked up in awe, "What's that?" he asked, His friend responded "That's an eagle, the king of birds. He belongs to the sky. We belong to the earth, we're chickens." So the eagle lived and died a chicken, because that's what he thought he was.

(Second Ending)

The eagle looked up in awe, "What's that?" he asked. His friend responded, "that's an eagle, the king of birds. He belongs to the sky. We belong to the earth, we're chickens." The eagle went through the day thinking of the eagle flying high. The next day the eagle went down to the pond. When he saw his reflection in the water, he noticed that he looked a lot like an eagle. He began to test his wings, flying further and further each day. After a few weeks, he was flying high and gliding just as if he were an eagle. Then he realized that he was an eagle. He was an eagle and not a chicken . . . With that thought, he flew above his past and his environment and so can you . . .

Chapter Twenty-Five
Insomnia

Everyone has had the experience at some time or another of tossing and turning for hours, re-adjusting pillows, sheets, and blankets, drinking hot milk or something stronger, or picking up a book and reading in hopes that it will put them to sleep. Though we have experienced this, most of us go to sleep easily most of the time. For those who constantly have trouble going to sleep, many things can cause insomnia: worry, guilt, fear, excitement over some upcoming event, reliving the events of the day. It seems that the more one tries to go to sleep, the wider awake one becomes. For the chronic sufferer, these problems are magnified many times over. Sleeplessness for them becomes the rule, not the exception, and their worry over not sleeping only compounds the problem.

(1) Mrs. Fontenot's Case History

Mrs. Fontenot, a 61-year-old woman, came to me because she was having trouble sleeping. She had been to a seminar which I lead on "Self Help With Self Hypnosis." This prompted her to come to me for counseling. Her safe place was a church and she always went there for the progressive relaxation. Mrs. Fontenot came to me for three sessions.

Using the finger response, I asked her the following questions:

1. Is there some emotional reason why you have difficulty going to sleep? *Yes.*
2. Does having difficulty going to sleep serve you some definite purpose? *Yes.*
3. Does worrying and thinking about problems prevent you from going to sleep? *Yes.*
4. Does your expectation of not going to sleep keep you awake? *Yes.*
5. Does your expectations of waking during the night keep you awake? *No.*
6. Does nervous tension keep you awake? *Yes.*
7. Does your inability to relax keep you awake? *Yes.*

8. Is there some inner conflict keeping you awake? *Yes.*
9. Are you identifying with someone else who had difficulty sleeping? *No.*
10. Are you using this problem as a means of punishing yourself? *Yes.*
11. Is there any sexual conflict that is keeping you awake? *No.*
12. Is there some past experience keeping you from sleeping? *Yes.*
13. Are you afraid you may have nightmares while you sleep? *No.* Is there any other reasons that you have trouble sleeping? *No.*
14. Is it OK with your subconscious mind for you to sleep easily and peacefully through the night? *Yes.*

During the regression, she went back to a time when she was angry with a nun. Mrs. Fontenot's favorite uncle who was a Methodist had died. The nun told her that because he was not a Catholic that he was going to hell. She responded, "No, and you are going to hell for saying that about my uncle. You are a witch. Look at that black robe, you are a witch. My uncle is in heaven." Of course, she was punished by the nun and again by her mother when she got home. Her father, whose brother had died, took her to the church. No one was there but the two of them. He consoled her and she felt comfortable, hence the church was her safe place. I explained to her that she could now look at that situation from an adult point of view. She was a little girl who loved her uncle. She could now be released from the need to punish herself. She was free now to go to sleep easily and comfortably.

(2) Overcoming Insomnia #1

You were born with the ability to sleep at any time you needed sleep. When you were a baby, you didn't think about sleeping or staying awake . . . When you needed sleep, you would automatically go to sleep . . . That's an ability you were born with, and that means it's an ability you still have . . .

You have the natural ability to go to sleep easily and quickly . . . When you desire to sleep, you can sleep even if it is noisy . . . You can sleep even if there is light in the room . . . And you can sleep comfortable regardless of your emotional state at the time when you go to bed . . .

There are many people who go to sleep almost as soon as they go to bed and you are just as capable of going to sleep quickly and easily . . . It keeps becoming easier and easier for you to relax and go into a deep sleep any time you desire to sleep . . . You can go to sleep just as easily as you did when you were a baby . . . You can go to sleep easily in any position, and in any surroundings . . . You can go to sleep even if it is noisy, and you can sleep comfortable even if there is light in the room or if it is totally dark.

Your subconscious mind has an amazing capacity for learning rapidly. Your mind already knows what to do to enable you to go to sleep quickly and easily, and can enable you to sleep comfortable and soundly . . . When you desire to sleep, you sleep normally, natural and awaken when it is appropriate for you to wake up or when someone wakes you . . . If something happens during the night while you are sleeping that makes it necessary for you to awaken, you awaken immediately and when you are ready to go back to sleep you are able to do so rapidly . . . You can sleep as long as you wish, and awaken at a time when you want to awaken . . .

Right now, you are relaxing in a hypnotic state, and you are learning that it is easy for you to relax and go to sleep and sleep peacefully and calmly . . . You have rapidly learned to go into a hypnotic state of relaxation, and you are realizing that it is just as easy for you to go to sleep anytime you go to bed for the purpose of sleeping. Whenever you want to go to sleep, you close your eyes and breathe deeply and exhale slowly seven times . . . Each time you inhale you feel yourself becoming drowsier, and each time you exhale, you continue becoming more relaxed. After breathing deeply and exhaling slowly seven times, begin counting backwards in your mind slowly from one-hundred . . . each time you try to think of the next number you continue becoming drowsier . . . and the numbers keep fading away, and soon disappear and you drift into a deep, peaceful sound, restful sleep . . . As you continue doing that each night, you automatically keep going to sleep more quickly . . . the numbers keep fading away more rapidly each time you use this method to go to sleep . . . and you always go into a peaceful, calm, restful sleep state as the numbers fade away . . . Each time you are ready to go to sleep, it keeps becoming easier . . . and it always is easy for you to awaken when it is time for you to awaken . . . During the day you feel more energetic, more cheerful and experience increased vitality . . . Your energy increases and your health continues improving more each day.

(3) The Waitress and the Little Boy

Earl Loonis tells of a little boy who went to a cafe with his mother and older sister. The waitress took the order of the mother and sister and then said to the little boy, "What will you have, young man?" His sister spoke, "I'll order for him." As if not hearing, the waitress repeated, "Young man, what will you have?" "A hamburger" the boy replied. "Would you like it rare, medium, or well done?" "Well done, please," said the boy. Would you like mustard, pickles, onions, relish, or ketchup?" With a smile on his face, he said, "The whole works!" As the waitress walked away, she heard the boy say, "Gee, Mommy, she thinks I am real."

Real life gives us a new self image which allows us to love ourselves. As a result of being affirmed by the waitress, the little boy was able to feel good about himself and affirm his own self-worth. When your dad took you to the church and consoled you, he was saying, "You are real. God loves you." You can now feel good about yourself. As you feel good about yourself, you are able to go to sleep easily whenever you desire.

(4) Overcoming Insomnia #2

Now you can let the cares of the day take care of themselves and enter into a peaceful, comfortable state of hypnosis. Sleep is a natural state for the body and the mind in order to re-energize, revitalize and heal. It is a natural gift that you give to yourself. First of all it is important to quit trying to go to sleep. Trying involves effort and effort, being a conscious process, tends to keep one awake. I'm certain you have heard many times that the harder you try to go to sleep, the wider awake you become. Sleep is such a natural state; all living beings sleep, but only people have trouble sleeping. That's because we are the only creatures who tries to go to sleep.

When you desire to go to sleep, assume a comfortable position lying down where you are not likely to be disturbed in a peaceful and quiet place. Take three deep breaths all the way down to your stomach and as you gently let out the first breath, give your eyes permission to relax and close. Focus your awareness on your eyes—allow them to relax even more. Relax them to a point that you are certain they won't open even if you wanted them to, because they are so relaxed and you want them to remain closed. Now allow that relaxation spread over your entire body, covering it like a soft, warm, fluffy blanket. Each time you do this, you find it progressively easier to relax deeply allowing your subconscious mind to make new positive associations each time and make relaxing and restful sleep an automatic and natural process for you. Now place your awareness on your breathing, causing you to go deeper and even deeper into relaxation. Focus on your abdomen and as you breathe in let your stomach expand and contract. Notice how it relaxes you more and more as you let loose of any of tightness or tension.

Now imagine your breathing sending oxygenated blood flowing through your body. Feel and imagine this oxygenated blood flowing now throughout your body and moving to the base of your spine . . . Then moving up the spine like mercury rises in a thermometer. Up the spine it moves to the neck, then to the tip of your head and then flowing to your forehead and back through your body. Picture and feel this oxygenated blood moving this way. Imagine as though it were water flowing down a creek carry away any points of tension in your body. With each breath you take, with each beat of your heart, with each blink of your eyes, feel yourself relaxing more deeply—feeling loose, limp and restful.

As you continue to inhale and exhale, notice the absence of tension. Your body and your mind reach a state of relaxation, calming, harmonizing. Your confidences in your ability is strengthening. You're feeling wonderfully good in each and every way. Each and every time you take a deep cleansing breath as you are now, this feeling of peace, serenity and calm fills your mind and body. All negative thoughts subside as if they are being washed away with each breath you take. Imagine your breathing dissolving all unwanted thoughts and tensions like a cube of sugar being dissolved in a cup of hot coffee. Watch it disappear. Feel it disappear. As you continue to go deeper and deeper with each gentle breath say to yourself, "I drift into a restful, peaceful, natural sleep. I sleep deeply and I awaken refreshed in the morning." Want it to happen. Expect it to happen. And let it happen.

Your powerful subconscious mind quickly releasing the conflicts for the day in order to release you from the stream of unwanted thoughts that prevent you from sleeping. Imagine yourself having a good day . . . Having all the resources both inside you and outside you to accomplish what you need to accomplish—realizing that life is a journey not a destination. Each moment relaxing making the next moment all that easier—feeling good about yourself—choosing a time to awaken tomorrow morning and waking and enjoying the new found energy you feel. Now continue to follow your breathing deeper and deeper into relaxation until you enter a gentle, sound state of sleep.

Tonight you let your relaxation carry you into a deep restful sleep from which you awaken in the morning totally refreshed. When you are ready to sleep (pause) sleep (pause) sleeping (pause) Deep sleep (pause) Gentle Sleep (pause) Calm (Pause) Refreshing Sleep (pause) Deeper,—

still deeper—and even deeper sleep. Take as much time as you need in the next one minute of clock time to let the suggestion sinking into your subconscious. During her last session, she reported that she was sleeping much better than she had in years. I concluded our last session with Blackboard Technique for Overcoming Insomnia.

(5) Blackboard Technique for Overcoming Insomnia

(Adapted from Marlene Hunter)

Imagine in your mind's eyes a blackboard; there is chalk there, and clean brushes. You pick up the chalk and a clean brush. You pick up the chalk in one hand and in the middle of the blackboard you put the number -1-, making it very nicely. That's right. Look at that for a few minutes, and then erase the -1- and up in the corner of the blackboard (I wonder which corner you'll choose?), up in the corner of the blackboard, you print the word "sleep" and you look at that for a time.

Now in the middle of the blackboard you put the number -2-, enjoying the feeling in your hand as you write that—nice, flowing lines—that's right. You look at that and then you erase it and up in the corner of the blackboard, again, you print the word 'sleep', and you look at that.

And in the middle of the blackboard you print the number -3-, I wonder how you'll make the -3-? With two half-circles, perhaps; I wonder if the upper one might be smaller or larger than the lower one, or the lower one smaller or larger than the upper one, so many different ways to make a the -3-. Look at the one you have chosen, then erase it and up in the corner, print the word 'sleep,' paying particular attention to the 'ee's' in 'sleep'—that's right.

Then in the middle of the blackboard you print the number -4-. Do you make the -4- with open lines or a closed triangle? There are so many different ways of writing -4-.

You continue this progression of printing a number and erasing it, and printing the word 'sleep,' and then another number and erase it, and so on. You are surprised to find yourself waking up in the morning! And it is always very interesting to think back on how many numbers you have written. It is very, very uncommon for people to have reached more than ten. You may be curious, if you decide to explore this particular approach; as to how many numbers you have written before you find yourself waking up this morning.

You know a lot about sleeping. Your body knows how to sleep—It has known how to sleep since before you were born! Let your body and your subconscious mind become reacquainted with that deep inner knowledge.

Your conscious mind, your thinking mind, can do whatever it wants to do; while your subconscious mind and your body renews this acquaintanceship. You may be aware of some of the warm, cozy feelings that the renewal evokes—you can be interested in those feelings, in your own awareness. Just let the feelings flow by, easily and gently, that's right. Tell your subconscious mind, and your body, that it is alright now to let that old, interrupted sleep pattern go, to be finished and put away, and that you now need a new, comfortable sleep pattern for the present, and for the future.. Enjoy the beginning of a new, useful pattern, and look forward to refreshing, restoring, replenishing, sleep every night.

Chapter Twenty-Six
Hypnosis in Sports

The use of hypnosis to enhance sports performance is widely recognized. Baseball, football, basketball, hockey, tennis players, bowlers, golfers, and other athletes practice hypnosis and self hypnosis to improve their performance.

An article in a 1984 issue of "Baseball Scene" reported that hypnosis helped the 1983 Chicago White Sox win the Western Division Championship of the American League. The White Sox hired Harvey Misel, a hypnotherapist, in mid-season to work with the team. Floyd Banister went from 3 wins-9 losses to 13 wins-1 loss for the rest of the season. Rich Dotson had a 13-2 record after working with Misel and ended the season at 22-7. Tom Paciorek batted .228 in the first half of the season and .320 for the second half. The White Sox went from third place in the American League West on July 1 to run away with the Western Division title. That same year Misel worked with Larry Bowa, Ron Cey and Bill Buckner of the Chicago Cubs and each showed a dramatic increase in their batting averages.

When asked how he helped, Misel stated that there have to be three common denominators present to succeed: the ability to concentrate will, confidence in abilities, and the ability to relax. Of course, hypnosis can not make one go beyond his abilities, but it can help the individual meet his potential.

The job of the hypnotherapist is to help the person remove negative mind sets which interfere with his skills and replace those negative thoughts with positive helpful thoughts. Sometimes a player is "trying" too hard and not doing what comes naturally: aiming his pitches, taking his eyes off the ball, and being too tense. A player can have great potential but if his mind is not in agreement, problems arise. The body will not do anything that the mind doesn't allow it to. By proper use of the mind, a player can live up to his abilities.

As you work with an athlete, understand that you cannot be completely familiar with all sports and every aspect of every sport. In order to help a player, you collect information from coaches or experts in the sport. With some knowledge in mind, determine areas where problems are experienced and make a plan to help the individual overcome the problem.

In addition to reaching relaxation, concentration, and self-hypnosis; positive suggestions and imagery are used. Imagery is very helpful and important in improving sports performance. The images should incorporate both seeing the necessary moves and experience the feeling of the muscles smoothly and easily following through with the visualization. Help the client translate his imagery into muscle movement as if he were doing it in reality. Emphasis is placed on doing it right, doing it just the way the client desires. A good suggestion is "You find that you easily keep your eye on the ball as it comes toward the plate, automatically estimating where the bat must be in order to accurately hit the ball. Feel your muscles following through automatically, enabling you to hit the ball." That statement works much better than "You won't strike out." You desire the client to focus on hitting the ball. Focus on the positive.

Self-Hypnosis is very important and can be used while actually playing the sport. The client can reinforce suggestions by use of post-hypnotic suggestion with a trigger mechanism. A batter may tap the plate and experience relaxed concentration. A pitcher may touch the bill of his cap and be focused for his next pitch. A golfer can take a deep breath and exhale slowly as he imagines where his next ball goes.

Have the client visualize himself doing the mechanics of his sport correctly. You may suggest, "Imagine you are succeeding at your sport. You are confident and in control, you see your actions and reactions as natural responses to the competition. You enjoy your sport and you succeed. You feel good about yourself and your confidence is increasing. Go through your mental rehearsal time and time again doing it just the way it should be done and have a positive attitude. You're mentally doing it just right."

(1) Joe Bob's Case History

Joe Bob, a 32-year-old man, came to me to help him enhance his performance in pistol competition. He had difficulty with his concentration and he was bothered by the noise of the crowd. As I knew little about pistol competition, I asked him to bring me some suggestions and imagery so that I could be more informed in my suggestions. I worked with him for three sessions and he increased his scores by 33%. I used "Self-Confidence" scripts, "Calm and Relaxed" script and my version of the information which Joe Bob had provided me.

(2) Pistol Competition Improvement

As you understand the course of fire, you feel sure of your abilities and have a positive attitude. You mentally rehearse what to do during the stage. As you prepare to shoot, you are relaxed and you are focused on what you're about to do . . . You are so focused on what you're doing in the competition. Noises and activities of the crowd only contribute to your relaxation and concentration . . . People talking, people watching only enhance your focus and concentration. Your thoughts are focused on the stage you are about to shoot and you have confidence in your ability to do it right . . .

As you assume the starting position, your body is relaxed, but you are ready to react instantly to the start signal. At the start signal, you draw your pistol and extend your arms toward the first target. Just as your arms are fully extended, the gun held firmly and you see the red dot on the target. The red dot is on the target every time you fire. You fine that red dot on the target when you pull the trigger. As you finish each position, immediately move quickly to the next position and just prior to moving there, start to extend the pistol toward the target so as you arrive, you are in the shooting position and the pistol is already extended toward the target. Shoot only as fast as you can see the red dot on the target. As you are focused, you quickly see the dot on the target.

During your mental imagery and before starting a stage, you plan how to shoot it. You know this before you start shooting . . . During planing of the stage, decide when to reload. When reloading, drop the magazine while at the same time taking a loaded magazine from you belt . . . Then tilt the pistol as you reload it. As soon as the magazine is locked in the pistol, you look up and bring the pistol on the target. Before the stage, you keep in mind that it is a Comstock Course or a Virginia Course . . .

You have complete alertness but remain relaxed and fluid. You focus on your abilities and let any other things going on around you contribute to your concentration . . . You do your best and you feel a sense of self-confidence that your best is good enough for you to compete successfully in the match . . . Picture yourself performing magnificently . . . Hitting the target and winning the match . . . Feel the good feeling of having done a good job . . . Rejoice in your improvement . . .

(3) Drew's Case History

Drew, a 21-year-old college baseball pitcher, came to me to help on his concentration while pitching. When pitching, he was at times brilliant and other times ineffective due to wildness. He would be pitching very good, lose his concentration and began to walk batters. When he lost concentration, the batters would begin to hit the pitches he threw across the plate. It was a vicious cycle which was blocking a promising future in professional baseball. I had seen him pitch many times and believed that he had great potential. I used a self-confidence script with emphasis on concentration and confidence while pitching. I told him that it was important for him to use his ability for imagery. He is to picture himself just as he wanted to be. I told him of the power of imagery to bring about his desires.

(4) Star Wars

One of the most popular movie series to come out in recent years has been the "Star Wars" movies. I would like to focus on the second one, "The Empire Strikes Back." Perhaps you saw that movie. If you did, nod your head "yes." He nodded "yes." (If "no," I say, "Well, let me tell you about it.") . . . You may remember in that movie, we continue with the heroes and villains of the first movie. Once again, we find ourselves engaged with Luke Skywalker, Hans Solo, Princess Lea, Chewbaca, and the robots R2D2 and C3PO, as they do battle with Darth Vader and the Legions of the Dark Empire.

One of the most fascinating new characters of "The Empire Strikes Back" is a strange little fellow named, "Yoda." The short, odd-looking little individual is the master teacher of the Jedi Knights. The Jedi Knights are commissioned as universal agents of goodness and righteousness.

Luke Skywalker is sent to Yoda for training to become a Jedi Knight, but the training does not always run smoothly. When Yoda attempts to teach Luke to raise Luke's space ship up and out of a swamp through the force of thought and imagery, Luke fails. After Luke's failure to move the ship, Yoda levitated the space ship up and out of the swamp by thought alone. Luke watches in amazement, saying, "I don't believe it!" Yoda responds, "That is why you failed."

The "Star Wars" movies are fictitious, but the story of Luke Skywalker and Yoda can be looked upon as a parable. Imagery is a powerful source of healing, overcoming unwanted habits, increasing self-confidence, and making positive changes in your life. Imagery consist of vividly picturing in your conscious mind desired goals, objectives, and holding that image until it sinks into your subconscious mind, where it releases great untapped energies. Imagery is based upon the principle that there is a deep tendency in human nature to ultimately become precisely that which one images himself to be. The wise old man of Proverbs states that whatsoever a person thinks in his heart, so is he. Jesus said, "Whatsoever you ask for in prayer, believe that you have received it and it will be yours."

(5) Pitching Concentration and Skills

You have told me that you have a desire to excel in your ability as a pitcher . . . You have chosen baseball as a sport in which you want to continue improving your talents, skills, and abilities. You love the game of baseball and have great enthusiasm for the game. You have the potential to be an exceptional and outstanding pitcher. And you have the talent and abilities to be an outstanding pitcher.

To be an excellent pitcher, the top players in the game say, there are several basic qualities and attitudes you must develop to help you be the outstanding player you are capable of becoming. You develop these qualities and attitudes and allow them to be planted into the soil of your subconscious mind which causes you to continually improve your abilities. You are becoming the outstanding pitcher you are capable of being . . . As I tell you those important qualities and attitudes, you can continue relaxing more completely and comfortable. You may find your mind wondering from time to time, but that is OK because your subconscious mind hears and receives everything I tell you and your subconscious mind allows these good suggestions to become your reality . . .

You have made a personal commitment to improve your skills and concentration. The desire to keep improving results in training and keeping your body in top physical condition at all times . . . You exercise your body regularly, practice to keep your body strong, fine tuned so that your reflexes and coordination always function properly. You eat the proper foods and avoid foods and drinks which diminish your abilities . . . Your desire to be an excellent pitcher continues increasing and that causes you to do the proper training needed to be an excellent pitcher . . .

A second quality in being an outstanding pitcher is to practice the skills of pitching correctly . . . Every sport requires that you have good speed, good timing, coordination, and the proper reflexes to enable you to make the right moves in the right way to handle your position properly . . .

It helps you improve your talents, skills, and abilities as a pitcher. You take some time each day to relax in a comfortable position and imagine yourself performing all the actions and techniques required for pitching. Imagine yourself doing everything properly . . . You do it correctly in your mind and that enables you to do it correctly when you are pitching in a game . . . Imagine yourself going over each pitch time and time again, always doing it properly. In an easy, natural way your mind directs your body to perform the moves and actions needed as you pitch.

Imagine concentrating on the catcher's glove and see the catcher's signal. In your mind, you see that ball going over the plate just where you want it to go and into the catcher's glove for a strike . . . You are relaxed and comfortable but with just enough adrenalin flowing in your body to respond appropriate to any situation. If at any time you become anxious or fear losing concentration step off the rubber, take a deep breath, touch the bill of your cap and as you exhale, you feel calm, relaxed and focused . . . You throw strikes or when attempting to fool a batter, you throw the ball where you want it to go . . .

A third quality to be an excellent pitcher is to be calm and at ease regardless of conditions or situations. You are increasing your ability and poise to adapt to any situation you are required to face . . . You pitch accurately whether the crowd is quiet or noisy, whether there are runners on base or not. Your concentration is focused under any condition when you are pitching. You are an outstanding pitcher and you have confidence in your abilities. You remain calm even if an error allows a man to reach base or when you walk an opposing batter . . .

When you are pitching, you are at your very best mentally, physically, and emotionally. You know by continuing to practice on the field and in your mind, you continue to improve. At any time you make a mistake, you accept it, learn from it, and maintain your concentration by stepping on the rubber, taking a deep breath, touching the bill of your cap and as you exhale, you are focused, relaxed and calm . . .

Drew was drafted by a professional baseball team and has been doing well in the minor leagues. His control has been excellent and his chances of moving up the ladder of his sport is good.

(6) Mr. Winegardner's Case History

Mr. Winegardner's is a retired business man who loves to play golf. He wants to be a successful golfer and has the talent to be good. The problem is that when he begins to play, he gets nervous and tense which reduces his abilities and effectiveness. I used the "Calm and Relaxed" script and "Building Self-Confidence" script with Mr. Winegardner. I concluded our session with a golf improvement script.

(7) Improving Your Golf Game

It is your desire to realize fully your skills and abilities to keep improving your golf game. You love the game of golf and have great enthusiasm for the game. It is your favorite activity of personal recreation, exercise, and competition . . . To be an excellent golfer, there are five basic qualities and attitudes which help you develop your skills to do your best. Knowing these qualities and planting them into your subconscious mind makes them increasingly real and beneficial to your golf game.

The first quality needed to improve your golf game is to experience an intense desire for the game. Your increased desire gives you a personal commitment to the game . . . Such desire manifest itself in training wisely and progressively to condition your body for this purpose. You know that to be a good golfer, you must practice and exercise appropriate skills. From now on, you are improving your ability to play golf by remaining calm and relaxed while you practice and play golf. Whenever you feel anxious or nervous, you take a deep breath, think of the words, "calm and relaxed," and as you exhale, you feel calm and relaxed, focused and ready to play with ease . . . You are properly motivated with the right attitude to reach your goal . . .

The second quality for excellence in golf is to correct any errors in techniques. You strive and find it easy to succeed in correcting all the techniques necessary to excel at golf . . . You employ your powerful imagination to picture and imagine yourself performing all the techniques in a manner you know is correct . . . You do it right in your imagination and you do it right when you are in competition with others . . .

The great golfer, Arnold Palmer said that imagination plays a great role in the game of successful golf. He said that most players have developed the ability to visualize the flight pattern of the intended shot. In visualizing, you subsequently produce a shot of similar projectory. Simply imagine for a few minutes that you are calm, relaxed and confident and imagine the type of shot you want to hit. As you come up to the ball continue to image just how it feels to hit the ball where you want it to go . . . Surprisingly, your mind directs your body to perform the moves that are needed for each stroke. From now on, you practice using your imagination and picture yourself doing what you inwardly want to do . . .

The third quality for excellence in golf is to be the master of your environment. When you play golf, you face various conditions. You increase your ability and poise to adapt to any situation with ease. You easily adapt to weather changes such as wind and rain or when the sun is bright or blocked by clouds. You adapt to different courses with comfort and ease . . .

The fourth quality for the best golfing is a competitive attitude. You welcome competition and you feel at ease in competition . . .

The fifth quality for good golf is that you dismiss all negative attitudes. Removing negative attitudes from your mind is highly important to your improvement in playing golf . . . Be convinced in your mind that you have the ability to play excellent golf. As you believe in your mind so it is . . .

You use your imagination both on and off the golf course. During your imagery, picture yourself calm, relaxed, and confident. Say to yourself, "calm and relaxed" and go on to play your game of golf in a calm, relaxed, confident, and winner manner . . .

Chapter Twenty-Seven
Dying and Death

During a seminar at Walter Reed Army Medical Center, Elizabeth Kubler-Ross (considered a pioneer in the study of dying and death), said, "It is hard to die, and it will always be so, even when we learn to accept death as an integral part of life, because dying means giving up life on this earth. But if we can learn to view death from a different perspective, to reintroduce it into our lives so that it comes not as a dread stranger, but as an expected companion to our life, then we can also learn to live our lives with meaning—with full appreciation of our finiteness, of limits on our time here."

Though we have begun to talk more about death, it is still a fearful frightening, happening. The fear of death is universal even if we think we have mastered that fear on many levels. Remember the words of Ecclesiastes 9:5, *"For the living know that they shall die."* Even though we accept the truth of that statement, we have difficulty in coping with our own feeling about death. To think of our own death is something we seldom do. I think it is important to come to some terms with our own dying in order to more effectively help those who are dying or those whose loved ones are in the process of dying.

I am going to give you five words. I would like for you to take a few minutes and give a short response to each word. Give your response in a word, a phrase, or no more that a sentence. Write down the first thing that comes to your mind. Following you can read my responses given the first time that I was asked to respond. There are no grades here, just give your answers. (1) Life, (2) Significant Others, (3) Unfinished Business, (4) Death, and (5) After Death. My responses:

1. Life: *Relationship.*
2. Significant Others: *People who have special meaning to me; family, friends, important religious and/or political leaders.*
3. Unfinished Business: *Mending of relationships that are important and getting business and personal affairs in order.*
4. Death: *End of relationships as I know them now.*
5. After Death: *New relationships—New beginnings.*

In working with the dying, one of the first questions of the doctor and the family is "to tell or not to tell." Though this is often the case, I feel that the question should be, "When to tell and how do I share this information with the individual?" If others know (staff, family members, friends), the patient will soon know even without being told and that may be a block to open communication. What are some of the problems caused by this game of denial? The failure to tell the patient sets up barriers because both the patient and others have to play games to keep from discussing the situation. Knowledge of the situation allows for better communicating and gives the patient a chance to complete unfinished business and more easily pass through the stages of dying.

Even though a patient is informed of the condition, I don't think a specific time should be given because some will die within the time phase just to keep the doctor from being wrong. Psychologically the patient may condition himself to die within the time given even though he may have lived longer or even overcome the disease if some hope were given. Though the situation should be open and honest, never take away the patient's hope. I believe that hope should always be available to the patient. I am sometimes asked about "false hope" and my response is that whether it is false hope or real hope, it helps the patient. No hope means death.

I remember a woman with leukemia who lived long beyond her expected death. The doctors encouraged her and often told her, "We are doing all we can and we hope for the best. Maybe some new medicine will be discovered that will reverse the destructive process of the leukemia." This was before I became involved with hypnosis but I did provide her with emotional and spiritual support. She was never given a time reference for her death and she maintained a basically positive attitude toward her situation. She once told me, "I could be depressed and bitter, but that would only hurt me, my family, and lower my resistance to leukemia." Hope gave her meaning as she tried to make the most of each day and her positive attitude gave her extra strength to fight her diseases. If she had not had hope, she would have probably had a much worse time and died sooner, so it would have done great harm to take hope from her. She realized that though she could not necessarily change her situation, she could choose what attitude she would take to her situation.

(1) Stages of Dying

When an individual has a terminal disease, there are usually five stages of dying (if time and situation permits) that one passes through. These are normal responses and therefore are not bad in themselves, but can become a problem, in one gets stuck in any of these areas. Each person may not follow the responses 1, 2, 3, 4, 5 and often some steps are skipped and at other times some steps are repeated. The Bible and modern psychology says experience those emotions and pass through them to new life and new faith.

1. *Denial and Isolation:* The main statements of this stage are, "Who me? No, not me, you have made a mistake. It can't be true. I want a second opinion. I'm sure there must be some mistake." Denial functions as a buffer after receiving unexpected and shocking news. It allows the patient to collect himself or herself and to begin mobilizing his or her resources to face the situation. Denial is usually a temporary defense but some maintain it for longer periods of time, some go back and forth and some never get beyond denial.

   The need for denial exist in every patient at times. It usually comes and goes and is usually followed by the patient's attempt to isolate himself from others. During periods of isolation, stick with the patient. When a person wants isolation, we tend to neglect and forsake them. Just be available.

2. *Anger:* When the first stage of denial cannot be maintained any longer, it often is replaced with anger, rage, envy, and resentment. The question changes from "Who, me?" to "Why me!" Because the patient may not know who to be angry with, they may show their anger toward family, doctors, nurses, chaplains, God, others, all. You may ask yourself, "How would I feel if all my life activities were to be so permanently interrupted?" Do you take the anger personally? By explaining the process to family members, you may be able to help family members better understand and accept the patient's anger.

   There was a man a Walter Reed Army Medical Center who was dying from an infection due to a stomach wound suffered in Vietnam. One day as I walked into his isolation room, he looked at me angrily and shouted, "Get the hell out of here you God damn Chaplain." I quickly left and as I shut the door I mentally said, "to hell with you." As I was stunned by the unexpected reception, I returned to my office. At that time I did not feel emotionally up to seeing any more patients. I began to think about the situation and how I should handle it. Should I quit visiting him, should I confront him about his verbal attack on me, or was there another way. After prayer and much thought, I decided that I did not want him to go to hell nor did I want to break off my relationship with him.

For the next five working days, I would go to his door, open it and say, "Hello John." and then close the door. On the sixth visit, I opened the door and said, "Hello John," but before I could close the door, he asked me to come in. After greetings had been exchanged, he told me that on the day of his verbal attack, his wife had told him that she was divorcing him. She would be returning to her home town and taking their two children with her. You see I happened to be the first person to visit him after she left so I received the brunt of his anger.

For a few, it is difficult to enter this stage. When it appears that one is holding back this feeling, I believe that they should be helped to express their feeling in non-destructive ways. The pain may be so great and the understanding so lacking, that the person wants to shake their fist at God and cry out, "Why! God! Why!" Many are afraid to do this for fear of making God angry and so suppress their hostility, doubt, and fear. From my experience as a hospital Chaplain, I have come to the conclusion that to properly express one's anger is a healthy reaction to the hurt one feels. I don't mean that one should let his or her anger out in destructive ways, but to discover what one is angry about and express it with someone they can trust.

If I am angry with someone but can't express it, a barrier is setup between me and that person that I am angry with. When we are able to talk about, the anger can be released and a more meaningful relationship can be established. The same is true when one is angry with God. In talking with God about my anger, I can let it go and a stronger faith can result. If I can't trust God to accept my anger, how can I expect God to accept me?

3. *Bargaining:* "If I can't get well by being angry, maybe I can make a bargain with God or fate for longer life." The question progresses from "Who me?" to "Why me!" to "Let's make a deal." Often the patient reverts to a childhood response. The child often makes demands, "I want . . . ," but when that doesn't work, he then reasons, "If I will be good can I?"

A Chaplain friend shared an incident which illustrates an unusual situation which occurred as a results of a bargain. The patient entered the hospital with symptoms of cancer which she had been cured of some five years before. Though she continued to lose weight, was suffering great pain, and losing strength, none of the test showed cancer. In the course of the Chaplain's visit, she told him that she had made a bargain with God during her last hospitalization. She asked God to allow her to see her youngest son through college and God had granted her wish because her son had graduated the previous May. The Chaplain helped her to accept the fact that God did not hold her to that bargain and that she was released from her part of the bargain which was her death. As she accepted this, she began to improve and in a few days was released from the hospital a healthy person in body, mind, and spirit.

4. *Depression:* When the patient can no longer deny because of her weakening condition, and neither anger nor bargaining have brought the desired results, she begins to feel a great loss. The question now becomes, "What's the use?" One comes to depression over the loss of certain activities and functions due to the illness and from the knowledge of the coming loss of life (preparatory grief). The person may not talk much, but needs and appreciates the presence of loved ones.

   I have found that guilt feelings may be a companion in any of the four stages of grief. If the patient sees illness and pain as a punishment for sin, he will try to determine what he has been done to cause the situation. If the patient can be helped to move through the guilt and experience forgiveness, they can experience great relief.

5. *Acceptance:* "I'm ready!" If given time and with some help, the patient will have been able to work through the previous stages. Acceptance should not be mistaken for a happy state, but may be void of much feelings. Few if any words may be exchanged, just be present so the person will not feel deserted.

Guidelines for working with a dying patient:

1. Be available and human
2. Allow the patient to set the pace
3. Accept the patient's anger
4. Offer yourself as willing listener
5. Do not abandon the patient
6. Respect the patient's individuality and protect his right to die with dignity.

(2) Mrs. Sharps' Case History

Mrs. Sharps, a 61-year-old woman, was in the hospital dying of cancer. She was alert, but losing strength and nearing death. The doctor consulted me for emotional and spiritual support. She was afraid to die because she felt guilty about something that had happened years before. Her friend had been harmed by some gossip which Mrs. Sharps had passed on to others. The friend had been dead for about three years. I had Mrs. Sharps imagine that her friend had come to the hospital to visit her. In the imagery, Mrs. Sharps was able to ask her friend to forgive her and the friend forgave her. Mrs. Sharps then asked God to forgive her and she felt and accepted God's forgiveness. I share with you two scripts which I used with Mrs. Sharps. She died in peace two days later.

(3) Light at the End of the Tunnel

I remember the story of a woman who wrote of her daughter's fear of tunnels as a child. As they traveled, the child would cling to her mother and press her face against her mother the moment they entered a tunnel. She would raise her head only after being assured that they had passed through the tunnel.

Several years later, they were traveling down the Pennsylvania Turnpike and approached a tunnel. The daughter had been gone from home for years, so her mother wondered how her daughter would react to the tunnel. As they traveled through the tunnel, the girl did not seem upset and maintained a pleasant attitude. The mother reminded her daughter of her childhood fear of tunnels, and asked her what brought about the change. The girl replied, "Mother, I found out that tunnels have light at both ends."

You now know that you have experienced forgiveness so you are aware that there is a light at the end of the tunnel.

(4) The Tree (by Audrey "Tucker" Morgan)

A little tree starts to grow in the country. It's right between its mother and father. As it grows up all the animals in the woods come to play around it. Soon it is tall enough that birds make their nest in it.

After years of growing, the woodsman come to chop down the tress. They look at the tree and decide to let it grow. The tree keeps growing, years go by. Still the tree keeps growing. People come in the spring and have picnics under the tree. It's branches make excellent shade for them. Years go by and the tree continues to get taller and taller. Now it is the tallest tree in the forest. Still it continues to grow.

After many years the tree grows beyond the clouds. One day it is growing and there around the tree's top branches is an opening into the heavens. There, looking down at the tree is God and his angels. God says, "We have been waiting for you!"

You see, no one told the tree how tall it could get. There were no limitations. You are now ready to grow beyond your limitations.

Chapter Twenty-Eight
Overcoming Grief

Ever since the day Adam and Eve bent over the body of their dead son, Abel, human beings have been suffering grief as a result of loss. Yet, in the full sense of the word, "grief," one can go back even further to the time when Adam and Eve ate the forbidden fruit and were expelled from the Garden, so in reality, grief goes back to that point in recorded history. Regardless of how you interpret the story of Adam and Eve, you have to acknowledge that human beings have been experiencing the gnawing, hurting, and painful experience over the loss of a valued object or person since the beginning of time.

Grief and the grieving process are not subjects you hear discussed often, so it's no wonder that one has trouble getting over grief. It has been said that while sex was the taboo subject of the first half of the 20th century, death has been the taboo subject of the second half. We continue to clothe death's reality with various phrases. Some of the phrases that come to mind are, "the deceased," "He expired," "She passed away," but seldom "He died."

"She died."

Some of the losses that can cause grief are:

1. loss of a mate by death, separation, divorce
2. loss of a parent or a child or a close friend
3. break up of an intimate relationship
4. moving from one place to an other
5. loss of pet
6. loss of opportunity
7. loss by crime
8. loss by accident or disaster
9. loss of wealth
10. loss of a body part; leg, arm, hand, breast
11. loss of self-image
12. loss of sexual ability
13. loss of self; anticipatory grief experienced by some with a terminal disease. Regardless of the cause of loss, a person may go through one or all of the stages of grief. Not all people go through all stages and there may be movement back and forth between the different stages.

Bereaved persons, faced with the death of a significant other show their feeling in various ways. A person may cry, stagger, feel weak, become nauseated, tremble, shiver, faint, hit a wall with his fist, or keep his or her emotions under rigid control. Different people will react in different ways.

(1) Stages of Grief

One of the first responses to the death of a significant other is that of shocked denial. "No, not John, you have made a mistake." "It just can't be, I was talking to him only an hour ago." "Mother is not dead, she is only sleeping." Denial is usually a temporary defense and is normal unless it is prolonged over a period of time.

An article in the newspaper carried this story, "Skeletal remains of a 78-year-old woman dead nearly a year, her skull resting on a pillow, have been found in a home shared by a daughter who continued living with the remains. Authorities said, 'The remains were discovered when the daughter's son came to visit his mother and grandmother.'" In correspondence, his mother referred to his grandmother being alive. This story reveals a case of prolong denial and morbid grief.

The denial stage maybe followed by crying and or almost empty feeling of shock. During this time, it is better to encourage the person to let their feeling be experienced. When we try to stop the crying, the hurt, the emotions, the individual may bury them deep where they can fester and eat away at the person causing problems months and or years later. Then when depression or other symptoms come, it is not connected with the interference of the grief process.

I visited a woman in the psychological ward at the American Military Hospital in Bangkok, Thailand who was scheduled for medical evacuation to the states. After we had talked for a while, she began to tell me about her mothers's death. She said that when she had been told of her mother's death, she began to cry. Her husband scolded her and said that Christians don't cry at death. She repressed her feelings and showed no more emotions toward her loss. After telling me this story, she seemed on the verge of tears. I told her to go ahead and cry, for Jesus blessed our mourning over the death of a loved one. She looked surprised and asked me to explain. I told her that Christ had cried when told that his friend, Lazarus, had died and in his beatitudes, he said, *"Blessed are they that mourn for they shall be comforted."* With that explanation, she began to cry. After her crying, she no longer had the nervous symptoms which had caused her hospitalization and was released from the hospital two days later.

This woman stopped the grief process and it made her sick months later. Let the person who has been told of the death of a significant other face the full pain of their loss for this is healthy. Because of the difficulty some people have in facing grief, it is a temptation for others to suggest for a doctor to provide a sedative. In most cases, I am against giving a sedative at this time. To give a person in grief a shot or pill to tranquilize them only slows down the grief process and is harmful in the long run. People should be able to let the hurt out so they can move beyond the grief.

The grieving process can be delayed, but it cannot be postponed indefinitely, for it will be carried out directly or indirectly. If it is not done directly at the time of the loss, it will be done later at much greater cost to the personality.

If not allowed to mourn at the time, it may come out months or years later as the woman mentioned earlier or as a man who is a close friend of mine experienced. A friend of the man died and when he came to visit the man's widow she said, "My husband loved you as he would his own son." Later that day as he shared this with me and a few close friends, he began to cry. He had had a strained relationship with his own father at the time his father died some ten years before so was unable to mourn. Though this man was close to the man who died, he was really mourning the death of his father. Through the death of his friend, he was able to finish some unfinished business with his father and mourn his death. Now he could say, "I am crying because of the death of my father." He could then accept his father as never before—accepting their differences without being angry.

In the grief process, there may be preoccupation with the dead loved one or an identification with him or her. In preoccupation, the person talks about the dead loved one—what they were like—how they lived—what they did together. In identification, the person in grief takes on some of the characteristics of the dead loved one—come to have a similar disease—takes over the business—acts in the manner of the dead loved one.

A man died a month after he and his wife had ended their marriage by divorce. The last few days of his life, his ex-wife was by his side. Even though he was unconscious, she continually told him how much she loved him. When he died, she went into extreme grief, which was triggered by guilt and/or love. Her husband's hobby was raising registered dogs which she had never liked. After his death this became her hobby and she devoted much time in caring for the dogs.

In a newspaper article written shortly after the death of Elvis Presley, Arthur J. Snyder states that there is a growing awareness that anxiety, depression, serious illness and even death may occur on the anniversary of the death of a loved one. Elvis's mother died at the age of 42 in the month of August. It is reported that Elvis never properly mourned his mother's death and therefore died during the month of her death and at the same age. The article by Snyder was titled, "Elvis' Sudden Death Triggered by Anniversary Reaction."

Another reaction of grief may be anger. The person may show feelings of anger, hostility, rage, envy, and resentment. This anger may be focused upon a specific person: doctor, nurse, another family member, Chaplain, the dead person, God, self, or some other person.

As the Chaplain approached a woman whose child had died, the mother cried out, "Why did God let this happen?" The Chaplain did not answer, but simply took her hand. She said, "I want to go somewhere and cry." The Chaplain responded, "Would you like to go to the Chapel?" "Just the opposite, I need to scream and rage at God. O God, Why did you let this happen to my child?" The Chaplain did not criticize her feelings nor did he try to defend God, but said, "You can do that too and perhaps it will help to have someone with you." He helped her release the tension and anger and move past the anger to readjustment.

"Why did he have to die on me?" Anger toward the person who died for having deserted the loved one. "If they had operated sooner." Anger toward the doctor. "You damn nurses are a bunch of sadists who enjoy seeing people suffer." Anger toward nurses. "If John would have brought mother to the doctor sooner, she would still be alive." Anger toward another family member.

Following anger, a person may go into a stage of depression. When the full reality of the death of a significant other floods one's life, he or she may begin to feel a sense of great loss. A woman's husband died and she withdrew from most of her social contacts. Though she had been very active in her church and several social clubs, now she seldom left home. Due to the caring love of a pastor and other members of her church, she was able to finally give up her depression and live a normal life.

Guilt is perhaps the most painful companion of death. "If only I had been there." "If I would have insisted on his going to the doctor." "If I had been a better husband/wife/father/mother/daughter/son!" "Why did I argue with her yesterday?" "It is all my fault." In a seminar at Walter Reed Army Medical Center, Edgar Jackson said, "It is accepted as established fact that all grief involves some guilt." It does little if any good to tell a person in grief that they should not feel guilty. You may help them through the guilt by listening and providing positive impute concerning their relationship.

As you work with people in grief, remember that it's healthy to cry, to express those deep feeling of anger and guilt that may accompany the loss. Let them talk about their feelings without being judgmental. If they are able to work through the grief process, they can emerge healthy throughout the experience. Granger Westburg once said that healing begins as the person passes through the grief process by starting to free himself from the bondage of the dead loved one, makes adjustments in the environment in which the loved one is missing. The person is now free from new relationships or patterns of interaction that bring rewards and satisfaction.

We who deal with people in grief can help the grief process be normal in many cases that would otherwise be abnormal. If we, as members of the helping professions, can help people in grief get "In Tune" with their feelings and begin the grief process, we can help the client avoid some unnecessary agony and suffering in the future. Occasionally you may have a client who has not properly mourned the death of a loved one. It is your job to help that person pass through the grief process and release any morbid grief.

(2) Mrs. Landry's Case History

Following the death of her husband, Mrs. Landry, a 32-year-old female, came to me for counseling. She said, "I just can't get over the death of my husband. I used to be active in the community, exercised four to six times a week, ate good, but now I don't go anywhere except to work, don't exercise, and don't eat properly. I don't like what I have become."

She blamed herself for her husband's death because she did not insist that he go to the doctor when he complained of chest pains. Upon questioning her, I discovered that he had complained of chest pains before that night, but would take a Rolaide and feel better after a short time. She felt that she could have been a better wife and then perhaps he would still be alive.

(3) Grandma Embroidering a Pillowcase

(Good for someone in grief or facing a baffling situation.) A number of things happen in life which are difficult to understand and certainly the death of a loved one is one of those things. St. Paul must have been thinking of these things when he wrote, *"Now we see through a glass darkly, but then face to face. Now I know in part, but then shall I know even as I am known."* These problems are indeed difficult to comprehend, for now we see only the baffling reflection in a mirror, but then face to face.

Our knowledge is sometimes limited and we do not have enough facts to pass judgement. As humans we often take the short view because we don't have all the facts. My grandmother used to embroider pillowcases and I remember as I sat at her feet watching her sew, there seemed to be no meaning or design to what she was doing. It was just threads crossed and re-crossed. Seeing that I was puzzled, she told me to come stand beside her so that I could see the pattern from her side. I did as she requested and as I looked at it from her view point, I saw a beautiful scene being sewn to perfection; thread by thread and strand by strand. It is often so with us in our view of life. We look at life from one side only, and from this side it often looks like a blotch of threads crossed and re-crossed in wild confusion. Until we are able to see life from both sides and have more facts at hand, we often see only the baffling reflection in a mirror.

(4) Stopping Too Soon

During the hypnotic session, I suggested that maybe she had stopped too soon in her grieving process so I told her this story:

Several years ago when the late Dr. Robert E. Goodrich was pastor of the First Methodist Church of Dallas, Texas, he and his family went on vacation. As it was late in the afternoon and several miles from the next city, they returned to the nearest town for the night. In the hotel cafe that night, they met some old friends who told them of one of the most beautiful sights that they could ever hope to see. After the friend had told them what highway to travel in order to see this wonderful sight, Dr. Goodrich responded that they had traveled that road and saw nothing outstanding. The friend asked, "How far did you go?" When he was told, the friend replied, "That's the trouble, you turned around too soon. Had you gone over the next ridge, you would have seen a sight that you could never forget."

The Goodrich's stopped too soon and therefore had no idea of what was beyond the other side of the ridge. So often in the midst of sorrow and grief, we are tempted to stop too soon, but need to go on to the comfort on the other side. Remember the words of Jesus in the beatitudes, "Blessed are they that mourn for on the other side of sorrow there is comfort." "Blessed are they that mourn for they shall be comforted" (Paraphrase of Matthew 5:4).

I then had Mrs. Landry imagine her husband sitting in a chair in front of her so she could talk to him and complete any unfinished business with him. I said, "Say what you want to your husband." She said, "Bill, I am so sorry that I did not go with you to your mother's that last weekend.

Please forgive me. I am sorry I didn't insist on your going to the doctor that night." She experienced his forgiveness for he said that he understood that she had a difficult week at work and just needed to relax for the weekend. He asked forgiveness for making a big deal of it and leaving to see his mother mad at his wife. He also reminded her that she had tried to get him to go to the doctor that night, but he refused.

I said, "You have been forgiven and have forgiven, now forgive yourself. As you forgive yourself, you are free from the need to punish yourself. You can begin to live a full life once again. You can be active in your community, exercise appropriately, eat well, and feel good about yourself." I concluded the session with "Overcoming Depression #2."

(5) Overcoming Depression #2

You have experienced the very painful loss of your husband and that can't be changed, but you can do something about it. You have a wonderful, almost magical transforming power within you, which can free you from inner fears, and can liberate you from your grief, misery, and frustration. This is the meaning of those words in the Bible, "You can be transformed by the renewing of your mind." As your mind is renewed, it brings harmony into your life, and the creativity of your mind responds accordingly. You have received and given forgiveness and so you are now able to renew your mind so that you can transform those negative feelings to positive helpful ones.

You are realizing that those feeling of depression were caused by thoughts, ideas, beliefs, opinions, theories, and the unpleasant experience of the death of your husband which has made a negative impression in your mind. But you are being changed by changing how your mind reacts to these things. You are releasing the tension and anxiety that have been in control for the past few weeks. You are continuing to relax even more now and you can do this in your daily life even when you experience stress, worry, or anxiety. Just take a deep breath and let the negativity out.

Regardless of where you are, or what you are doing, your find that more and more, day by day, you are more calm and relaxed, and are able to cope with your every day changing circumstances. Your self-confidence, self-esteem, and self-worth are increasing each day.

You are understanding that you are a spiritual being, created by God. As a spiritual being, you have intelligence and wisdom that can release you from all anxiety and confusion. You trust the love and goodness of God to help you through each and every day. You feel the goodness of God setting you free from all mistakes of the past. The love of God is releasing you from all guilt and is cleansing your mind, soul, and body. You are beginning to feel a pure stream of God's love flowing through you; cleansing, healing, purifying, and restoring your joy and motivation for living. You feel your body being strengthened and renewed with energy, vitality, and enthusiasm.

Each day your self-confidence keeps increasing and you continue living your life with a greater feeling of poise, peacefulness and joy. You are open and receptive to all the good things available to you in life. You are filled with a sense of well-being and joy.

Conclusion

I believe that great times are ahead of us for the use of hypnotherapy. In order to fulfill our potential, we must work together. We can best fulfill our potential by respecting, uplifting, and learning from one another. To put another hypnotherapist down is unproductive and detrimental to all hypnotherapists. A Rabbi once asked his pupils, "How can you tell when the night had ended and the day was dawning?" "Could it be when you can see an animal at a distance and can tell whether it is a sheep or a dog?" asked one student. "No." said the Rabbi. "Could it be when you can look at a tree in the distance and tell whether it's a fig tree or a peach tree?" "No." said the Rabbi. "Well, when is it?" demanded the students. "It is when you look on the face of a woman or man and see that she or he is your sister or brother because, if you cannot do this, then no matter what time it is, it is still night." Jesus said, "A house divided by itself cannot stand" (Mark 3:25).

There is a story about a man who left this earth and was taken on a tour of hell. He was shown a room where he saw a large group of hungry people trying to eat dinner, but because the spoons that they were using to eat with were longer than their arms, they remained frustrated. "This," his guide told him, "is hell." "That's terrible!" exclaimed the man, "Please show me heaven." "Very well," said the guide, and they went on their way. When they opened heaven's door, the man was perplexed to see what looked very much like hell. There was a group of people with spoons longer than their arms. As he looked more closely, however, he saw happy faces and full stomachs, for there was one important difference. The people in heaven had learned to feed each other.

There are mountains to climb and rivers to cross, but we are making advances which will be of great benefit to the people of our world. Let us accept the challenge in unity and begin to climb the mountains and cross the rivers as we fulfill our mission.

As hypnotherapist, our mission is to kiss frogs. We do that by the proper use of suggestions, imagery, and healing stories so that the client can become a prince or princess. There are many froggish people who feel slow, low, ugly, drooped, and pooped. They seem to be floating aimlessly on their lily pads needing a symbolic kiss. Other frogs are puffed up in their own little world. They appear to be successful and on top of the world, but inside there is a lack of meaning and a feeling of inner emptiness. They too need to be symbolically kissed. It is great to see a frog turn into a prince or princess so go on kissing frogs.

BIBLIOGRAPHY

Adams, P. (1967). *The New Self Hypnosis.* Hollywood, CA: Wilshire Book Company.

Ansari, M. (1982). *Modern Hypnosis.* Washington, D.C.: Mas-Press.

Atwood. C., & Atwood, S. (1990). *Scripts You Can Use.* Phoenix, AZ: Atwood Institute of Research and Education.

Barnett, E.. (1979). *Unlock Your Mind and Be Free.* Glendale, CA. Westwood Publishing.

Barnett, E. (1989). *Analytical Hypnotherapy.* Glendale, CA. Westwood.

Beveridge, I.C. (1992). *Hypnotherapy: Its Christian Aspect.* Columbus, GA: Brentwood Christian Press.

Beveridge, I.C. (1995). *Induced to Produce.* Columbus, GA: Brentwood Christian Press.

Bolduc, H.L. (1992). *Self-Hypnosis.* Virginia Beach, VA: ARE Press.

Boyne, G. (1982). *Hypnosis: New Tool in Nursing Practice.* Glendale, CA: Westwood Publishing.

Brigham, D. (1994). *Imagery for Getting Well.* New York: W.W. Norton.

Bryan, W.J. (1988). *Religious Aspects of Hypnosis.* Ann Arbor, MI: Access Information.

Cage, R. (1984). *Conflict Therapy Hypnotherapy.* Fort Worth, TX: Mental Dynamics Institute.

Caprio, F.S., & Berger. J.R. (1963). *Helping Yourself With Self Hypnosis.* Englewood Cliff, NJ: Prentice-Hall.

Caprio, F. (1985). *Better Health with Self Hypnosis.* New York: Parker Publishing.

Coffey-Lewis, L. (1982). *Be Restored to Health.* New York: Ballantine Books.

Cook, C.E. & Van Vogt. (1956). *Hypnotism.* Alhambra, CA: Borden Publishers.

Copeland, R. (1981). *How to Hypnotize Yourself and Others.* New York: Barnes & Noble.

Cunnigham, L. (1981). *Hypnosports.* Glendale, CA: Westwood Publishers.

Durbin, P.G. (1993). *Human Trinity Hypnotherapy.* Ann Arbor, MI: Access Information.

Elliot, R. (1991). *Wide Awake, Clear-Headed, and Refreshed.* Winfield, IL.: Relaxed Books.

Elman, D. (1977). *Hypnotherapy.* Glendale, CA: Westwood Publishing.

Erickson, M. (1982). *My Voice Will Go With You.* New York: W.W. Norton.

Fanning, P. (1988). *Visualization for Change.* Oakland, CA: New Harbinger Publishing.

Farago, R. (1993). *Hypno Health.* London, England: Vermillion.

Fegler, W. (1980). *Just Imagine.* Hollywood, CA: Laurida Books.

Fisher, S. (1991). *Discovering the Power of Self-Hypnosis.* New York: Harper Perennial.

Frances, C. (1993). *Counseling Hypnotherapists.* Merrimack, NH: NGH.

Frances, C. & Hughes J.C. *Scripts and Tips.* Merrimack, NH: NGH

Francuch, P. (1981). *Principle of Spiritual Hypnosis.* Santa Barbara, CA: Spiritual Advisors Press.

Friedman, E.H. (1990). *Friedman's Fables.* New York: Guilford Press.

Gagnon, L. (1986). *RX: Hypnosis.* Leo Gagnon.

Gaines, B. (1991). *New Concepts of Hypnosis.* Hollywood, CA: Wilshire Book Co.

Hadley, J., & Staudacher, C. (1955). *Hypnosis for Change.* Oakland, CA: New Harbinger Publishers.

Hammond, D.C. (1990). *Hypnotic Suggestion and Metaphor.* New York: W.W. Norton and Co.

Havens, R., & Walters, C. (1992). *Hypnotherapy for Health, Harmony, and Peak Performances.* New York: Brunner/Mazel.

Havens, R., & Walter, C. (1989). *Hypnotherapy Scripts.* New York: Brunner/Mazel ("Protective Ants" p. 132 and "Inside Barrier" p. 141 reprinted by permission.).

Henderson, C.E. (1983). *Self Hypnosis.* Englewood Cliff, NJ: Spectrum Books.

Hilgard, E., & Hilgard, J. (1975). *Hypnosis in the Relief of Pain.* Los Altos, CA: William Kaufman.

Hughes, J.C. (1990). *Hypnosis: The Induction of Conviction.* Hollis, HN: Transcendental Publications.

Hunter, M. (1988). *Daydreams For Discovery: A Manual for Hypnotherapists.* West Vancouver, B.C. (Canada): Sea Walk Press.

Hunter, C.R. (1994). *The Art of Hypnosis.* Merrimack, NH. NGH.

Hunter, C.R. (1995). *The Art of Hypnotherapy.* Dubuque, IA: Kendall/Hunt Publishing Company.

Kappas, J.G. (1975). *Professional Hypnosis Manual.* Panoroma City, CA: Panorama Publishing.

Kelly, S., & Kelly, R. (1985). *Hypnosis.* Reading, MA: Merloyd Lawrence Books.

Korn, E.R. & Johnson, K. (1983). *Visualization: The Uses of Imagery in the Health Professions.* Homewood, IL: Dow Jones-Irwin.

Krasner, A.M. (1990). *The Wizard Within.* Santa Ana, CA: American Board of Hypnotherapy Press.

Kresnik, J.J. (1988). *Hypnotherapy Scripts.* Vol. I & II. Denver, CO: Hypnotherapy Institute of Colorado.

Kroger, W. (1977). *Clinical and Experimental Hypnosis.* Philadelphia, PA: J.B. Lippencott Co.

Lankton, C., & Lankton, S. (1989). *Tales of Enchantment.* New York: Brunner/Mazel.

Lagarus, A. (1985). *In the Minds Eye.* New York: Guilford Press.

LaVille, J. and S. (1994). *101 Hypnotic Suggestions.* Bonito Springs, FL: IACT.

LeCron, L. (1964). *Self-Hypnosis.* New York: Segnet.

Levine, B. (1991). *Your Body Believes Every Word You Say.* Bolder Creek, CA: Aslon Publishing.

Longacre, R.D. (1995). *Client-Centered Hypnotherapy.* Dubuque, Iowa: Kendall/Hunt Publishing Company.

Longacre, R.D. (1995). *Visualization and Guided Imagery for Pain Management.* Dubuque, Iowa: Kendall/Hunt Publishing Company.

Longacre, R.D. (1989). *Inside Out: Pathway to Change.* Glendale, AZ: Therapeutic Education.

Longacre, R.D. (1990). *Practical Therapies for Catastrophic Illness.* Glendale, AZ: Therapeutic Education Group.

Lusk, J. (1992). *30 Scripts for Relaxation, Imagery, and Inner Healing, Vol. 1.* Duluth, MN: Whole Person Associates.

Lusk, J. (1993). *30 Scripts for Relaxation, Imagery, and Inner Healing, Vol. II.* Duluth, MN: Whole Person Associates.

McGill, O. (1987). *Power Hypnosis Hypnotherapy.* Merrimack, NH: NGH.

Meyers, R.G. (1992). *Practical Clinical Hypnosis.* New York: Lexington Books.

Middleton, N. (1993). *Imaginative Healing Using Imagery.* Saratog, CA: R & E Publishers.

Miller, R. (1993). *Your Unlimited Potential.* Monteclair, NJ: Unlimited Potential.

Mills, J., & Crowley, R.J. (1986). *Therapeutic Metaphors for Children and the Child Within.* New York: Brunner/Mazel.

Morton, R. (1980). *Hypnosis and Pastoral Counseling.* Los Angeles, CA: Westwood Publishing.

Murphy, J. (1982). *The Power of Your Subconscious Mind.* New York: Bantam Books.

Osborne, C. (1973). *The Art of Understanding Yourself.* Grand Rapids, MI: Zondervan.

Parker, W.R., & St. Johns, E. (1957). *Prayer Can Change Your Life.* New York: Prentice-Hall.

Peale, N.V. (1985). *Positive Imagery.* New York: Faucett Cress.

Petrie, S., & Stone, R. (1981). *Hypno Cybernetics.* New York: Parker Publishing.

Pratt, G., & Wood, D., & Almon, B. (1988). *A Clinical Hypnosis Primer.* New York: John Wiley and Sons.

Rosen, S. (1982). *My Voice Will Go With You: Teaching Tales of Milton Erickson.* New York: W.W. Norton.

Rossi, E. (1986). *The Psychology of Mind-Body Healing.* New York: W.W. Norton.

Rossman, M. (1989). *Healing Yourself.* New York: Pocket Books.

Shrout, R.N. (1985). *Modern Scientific Hypnosis.* North Hamptonshire, England: Thorson Publishing Limits.

Simonton, C., & Simonton, S., & Creighton, J. (1978). *Getting Well Again.* New York: St. Martin Press.

Sparks, L. (1961). *Self Hypnosis.* Hollywood, CA: Wilshire.

Stiles, W. (1994). *How Hypnotherapy Can Help.* Dubuque, Iowa: Kendall/Hunt Publishing Company.

Stormer, M. (1992). *Hypnosis Handbook.* Dallas, TX: Hypnosis Institute of Texas.

Tibbits, C. (1977). *Self Hypnosis.* Glendale, CA: Westwood Publishing Company.

Van Nostrand, R. (1991). *Metaphor Magic For Treating Co-dependency.* Tulsa, OK: Van Nostrand.

Wagner, J.K. (1992). *Healing Ministry of Christ in the Church Today.* Nashville,TN: Upper Room Books.

Waldrop, C.S. (1989). *Getting Good at Being You.* Nashville, TN: Broadman Press.

Wallas, L. (1985). *Stories for the Third Ear.* New York: W.W. Norton ("Green Dragon" used by premission of W.W. Norton & Company, Inc. Copyright © 1985).

Wester, W., & O'Grady, D. (1991). *Clinical Hypnosis with Children.* New York: Brunner/Mazel.

Wheatherhead, L. (1951). *Psychology, Religion, and Healing.* Nashville, TN: Abingdon Press.

Winkler, A. (1990). *Hypnosis: A Key to Health, Happiness and Success.* Springfield, LA: St. John University Publications.

Winkler, A. (1989). *Hypnotic Inductions and Prescriptions.* Springfield, LA: St. John's University Publications.

Wright, M.E., & Wright, B. (1987). *Clinical Practice of Hypnotherapy.* New York: Guilford Press.

Yapho, M. (1990). *Tranceworks.* New York: Brunner/Mazel.

Zeig, J. (1990). *A Teaching Seminar with Milton Erickson.* New York: Brunner/Mazel.

Zilbergild, B., & Edstein, M.G. (1986). *Hypnosis Questions and Answers.* New York: W.W. Norton.

AUDIO-VISUAL BIBLIOGRAPHY

Atwood Institute for Research and Education. *Hypnotherapy Course* [36 videotapes]. Phoenix, AZ.

Bauer, L. *Seminar on Subconscious Mind* [2 Videotapes]. Slidell, LA.

Cousins, N. (1984). *Mind Over Illness* [6 audiotapes]. Chicago, IL: Nightengale-Conot.

Elman, D. *Course in Clinical Hypnosis and Hypnotherapy* [36 Audiotapes). Glendale, CA: Westwood Publishing.

Erickson, M. *Exploration In Hypnosis and Therapy* [videotape].

Hypnosis Motivation Institute. *HM 101, 201, 301* [18 videotapes]. Tarazano, CA.

Kein, G. *Pain Control Techniques, How to Conduct a Lecture, Hypnotic Techniques for Male Impotence, and Hypnosis for Fear and Phobias* [4 videotapes]. Fort Lauderdale, FL: Omni Hypnosis Center.

Long, T. (1978). *Professional Hypnotist Seminar* [10 audiotapes]. Automated Learning.

Longacre, R.D. *Hypnotic Anaesthesia* [2 videotapes]. NBHA.

Maltz, M. (1989). *Psycho-cybernetics* [8 audiotapes]. Irvindale, CA: Guthy-Renher.

McGill, O. *Applied Hypnosis (volumes 1, 4, 5)* [videotape]. Santa Rose, CA: Hypnotherapy Training Institute.

Peale, N.V. (1982). *Positive Thinking* [6 audiotapes]. New York, NY: Positive Communications.

Pulos, L. (1993). *The Power of Visualization* [6 audiotapes]. Niles, IL: Nightengale-Conant.

Reel, J. (1981). *Vanguard Techniques* [videotape].

Siegel, B. (1986). *An Evening with Bernie Siegel* [videotape]. New York, NY: Upstate Medic.

Sontged, A. (1980). *Hypnotism Workshop* [6 audiotapes]. Self-development Research.

Spencer, A. *Hypnotherapy Course 1 and 2* [16 audiotapes]. Royal Oak, MI: Infinity Institute.

Spiegel, H., & Spiegel, D. (1982). *Clinical Hypnosis* [16 audiotapes]. Gilford.

Van Fleet, J. (1994). *Subconscious Mind Power* [6 audiotapes]. Niles, IL. Nightengale-Conot.

Winkler, A., & Winkler, P. *Hypnotherapy Course* [44 Videotapes]. Springfield, LA: St. John's University.

Wood, T. *Rapid Inductions in the Medical Setting* [1 audiotape]. Tucson, AZ: Hypnosis Training Institute.

Zelling, D. *Post Graudate Course in Practical Hypnosis* [8 audiotapes]. Ohio Institute of Medical Hypnosis.

Zelling, D. *Pain Management* [4 audiotapes]. Ohio Instutite of Medical Hypnosis.

Zelling, D. *Human Sexuality* [9 audiotapes]. Ohio Institute of Medical Hypnosis.

Zelling, D. *Sports Hypnosis* [4 audiotapes]. Ohio Institute of Medical Hypnosis.

Zelling, D. *Treatment of Depression* [8 audiotapes]. Ohio Institue of Medical Hypnosis.